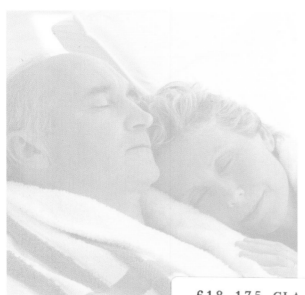

Hormones or Natural Alternatives ?

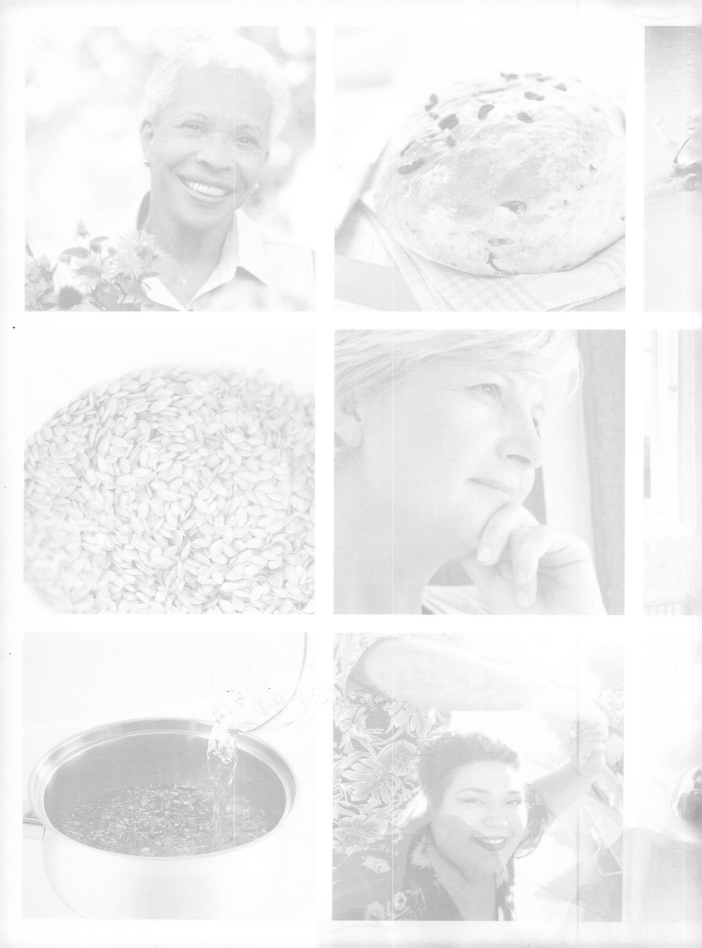

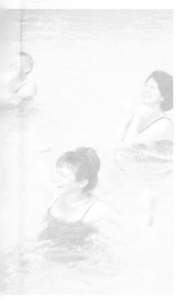
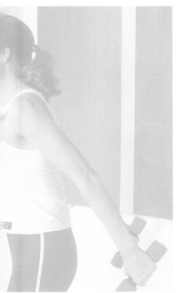

Hormones or Natural Alternatives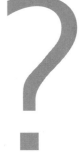

JAN CLARK

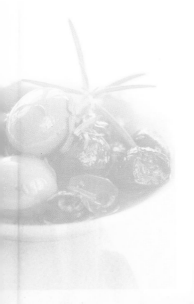

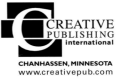
CREATIVE PUBLISHING international

CHANHASSEN, MINNESOTA
www.creativepub.com

First published in the USA in 2003 by
Creative Publishing international, Inc.

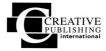

18705 Lake Drive East
Chanhassen, Minnesota 55317
1-800-328-3895
www.creativepub.com

President/CEO: Michael Eleftheriou
Vice President/Publisher: Linda Ball
Vice President/Retail Sales: Kevin Haas

First published in Great Britain in 2003 by
Hamlyn, a division of Octopus Publishing
Group Ltd, 2–4 Heron Quays, London E14 4JP

ISBN 1-58923-106-6

Printed and bound in China
10 9 8 7 6 5 4 3 2 1

SAFETY NOTE

While the advice and information in this book
are believed to be accurate and true at the
time of going to press, neither the author nor
publishers can accept any legal responsibility
or liability for any errors or omissions that
may be made. The reader should always consult
a physician in all matters of health and
particularly in respect of any symptoms which
may require diagnosis or medical attention.

Contents

Introduction

Few areas of women's health stir up as much confusion and debate as hormone replacement therapy or HRT, which arouses both condemnation and enthusiasm in equal measure.

The vast majority of women who are likely candidates for HRT are at a time in their lives when their hormones are in decline—between the ages of 50 and 60. What could be more natural than to 'pop-a-pill' to alleviate their menopausal symptoms, rejuvenate their middle years, and ensure a healthy old age? For there has been such an improvement in the quality of women's lives that the proportion of women living past the age of menopause has tripled during the past century, and is expected to increase steadily in the foreseeable future.

If adulthood is defined as beginning at the age of 21, the average age at natural menopause is 51 and the average life expectancy is 81, then women in the United States, in Europe, and in much of the developed world will live one-half of their lives in the years after menopause, a time of relative estrogen deficiency compared to their reproductive years.

The impact of this deficiency on some of our lives is so dramatic that we look for a medication to relieve its symptoms, and hormone replacement therapy may well be suggested by our doctors.

It should be a straightforward decision. But our hormonal patterns are as individual to us as our fingerprints, and it is not possible that the same hormonal preparation will suit every woman. Not only that, but for all its possible benefits, HRT carries potential risks.

Is it really possible for doctors to enhance a woman's quality of life by prescribing a medication and also to tell them this medication has some risks outweighing the benefits?

The confusion is fuelled by the media when it reports the latest research into some aspect of HRT which appears to contradict previous findings. Furthermore, few doctors suggest natural alternatives to their patients: while some such natural remedies make dubious claims, others have gained a respectable track record of effectiveness, and are available from pharmacies, an increasing number of health food outlets and company websites.

This book sets out to present the facts and fiction about both hormone replacement therapy and its natural alternatives. Threading through the chapters are 'personal profiles' of women who have written to me about their experiences of both. Once you have read the book, you will be able to create your own 'personal profile' and thus make an informed choice about a decision that could affect the rest of your life.

I hope you will share this book with someone close to you.

Headaches, depression and anxiety can be unsettling during your menopausal transition.

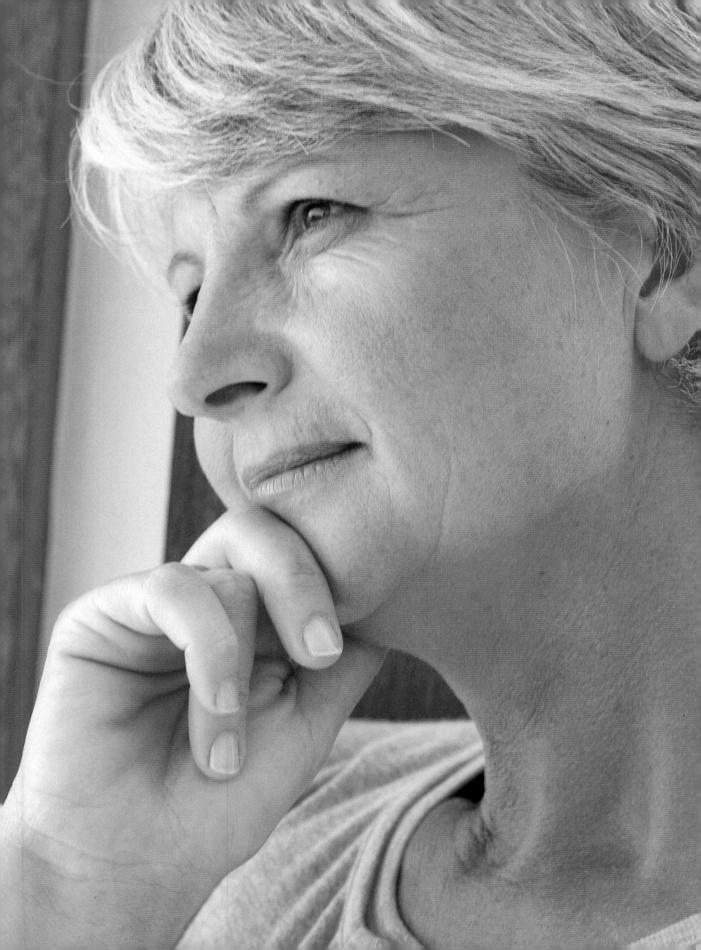

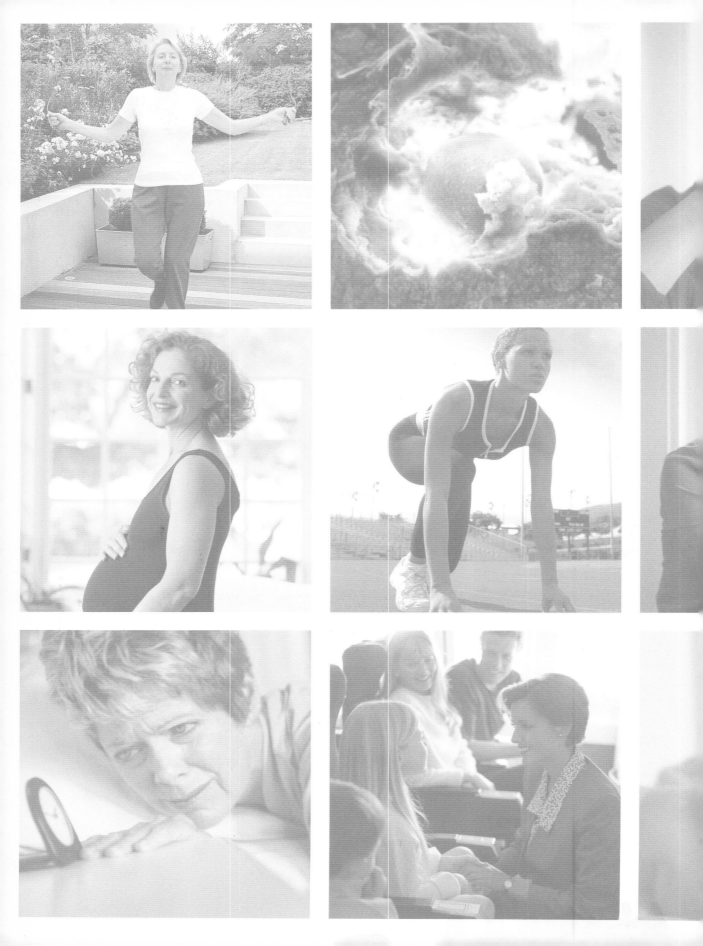

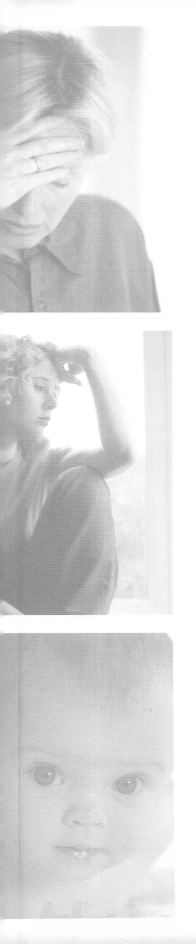

1

Hormonal
highways

Hormones and your body

Perhaps you have picked up this book because your doctor has recommended hormone replacement therapy (HRT) for your menopausal symptoms, saying that the hot flashes and dreadful night sweats which have troubled you for the past few weeks will vanish. What a relief that would be! Nevertheless, you have decided to find out more about it before committing yourself.

Or maybe you have been advised to undergo a hysterectomy, and the surgeon wants to remove your ovaries at the same time. The doctors say they serve no useful purpose now that you are menopausal, and the words "ovarian cancer" have been mentioned. As you have completed your family, you are quite happy to follow this advice. In passing, your physician has mentioned that you should take HRT after the operation. This has alarmed you because your sister takes it and has gained a huge amount of weight. You wonder if this will happen to you.

Or perhaps you found yourself bursting into tears one day at work when your boss commented on your lack of concentration. It's true that your memory has not been as razor-sharp as usual. As you later told the doctor, you are also sleeping fitfully and have no interest in sex. Your doctor thinks your symptoms are caused by menopause and recommends HRT as the solution. But you do not want to take it; you are sure there are other, perhaps more natural, ways to deal with your present situation.

Or possibly you are a young woman whose whole life is ruled by the agony of endometriosis. Every conventional drug available has failed to provide long-term sustainable relief. Surgery is now the only option, but this will entail removal of your ovaries and means you will never have children. You are likely to experience your menopause within two years. Your physician has recommended HRT after surgery as the only way to alleviate the symptoms. You are baffled about replacing your own hormones with manufactured ones, so you have resolved to find out more about HRT.

Or you are in your late 60s and, while in a cardiac rehabilitation unit at a hospital following a heart attack, have agreed to take part in a clinical trial of low-dosage HRT. The improvement in your life has been dramatic. You feel more energetic and lively than you have for years, and sexual intimacy has again become pleasurable now that your vagina is moist and soft. But a nagging anxiety disturbs your happy frame of mind. Your mother died of uterine cancer when she was 75, and you want to know more about the risks if you continue with HRT.

You may have been surprised to read the scenarios above, having thought that HRT is relevant only when a woman is in her 50s and menopausal. What they reflect is how our lives are continually influenced by our own particular "hormonal highways" at different stages of our lives. The influences of different hormones become more prominent as circumstances change.

Taking time to pause and reflect on changes in your emotional and physical life can be very helpful.

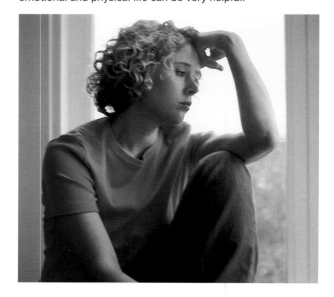

The endocrine system

Hormonal highways develop through the endocrine system—a number of glands that produce hormones. Endocrine glands work as a team and include:

- **The pituitary** Located at the base of the brain, the pituitary is responsible for the secretion of two hormones essential to the reproductive system: follicle-stimulating hormone (FSH) and luteinizing hormone (LH). The main activity of the pituitary is the control of the other endocrine glands.

- **The thyroid** Consisting of two lobes, one either side of the trachea (windpipe), the thyroid produces two hormones essential for normal metabolic processes and mental and physical development: T3 and thyroxine, or T4. T3 has a role in influencing mood and emotion, but its primary role is an accelerator of metabolism in all organs of the body.

- **The parathyroids** Usually four in number and found on the back and side of each thyroid lobe, the parathyroids produce hormones that increase the amount of calcium circulating in the blood.

- **The adrenals** These consist of a flattened body above each kidney and are made up of a cortex and a medulla. The adrenal cortex produces several hormones, including cortisol (which is important in carbohydrate breakdown and in the normal response to stress) and the sex hormones (estrogens and androgens). In men, androgens have an important role in stimulating the development of the sex organs, and the principal source of these hormones is the testes. However, androgen hormones produced by the adrenals also have a vital role in women. After the

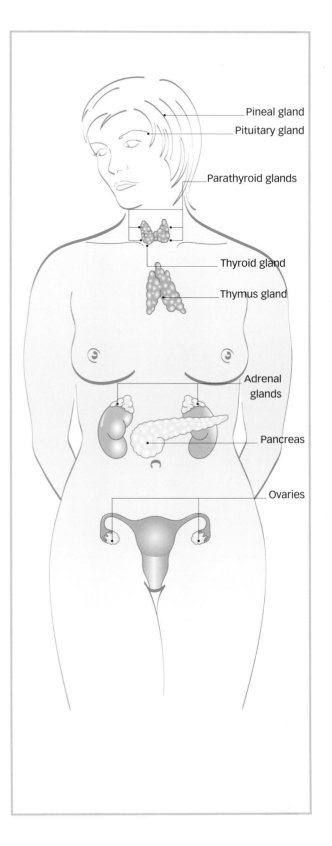

Pineal gland
Pituitary gland
Parathyroid glands
Thyroid gland
Thymus gland
Adrenal glands
Pancreas
Ovaries

menopause, some androgens, such as dehydroepiandrosterone (DHEA) and androstenedione, can be converted by the adrenals into estrone, a weak estrogen. This becomes the body's main source of estrogen when the ovaries have stopped producing it. The adrenal medulla secretes adrenaline (epinephrine) involved in the "flight or fight" response when in danger or under emotional or physical stress. A slow, rather irregular release of adrenaline goes on all the time, but any situation fraught with fear or anger significantly boosts production. When that happens, adrenaline increases the blood flow to the muscles by accelerating the heart rate and shutting off the less essential blood flow to skin and intestines.

- **The pancreas** This gland, which is located near the stomach, produces insulin, the hormone that regulates the level of sugar in the blood. Insulin allows glucose to enter the cells, where it is used as fuel.

- **The ovaries** In addition to producing eggs, the ovaries produce the hormones estrogen and progesterone (in response to FSH and LH from the pituitary gland) and testosterone.

What are hormones?

The word hormone comes from a Greek word *horman*, meaning "to stir up or arouse to activity", and this is exactly what hormones do. These chemical substances are made in minute quantities in glands and circulate around the body via the bloodstream. Each one has a specific effect on its target organ or tissue through controlling, activating, and directing structures and functions. Many hormones affect the urges, desires, and feelings that belong to you and nobody else. Hormone levels fluctuate throughout your life, influencing your moods, activities, and sensitivities as they ebb and flow.

Hormones also:
- Affect metabolic rate (how quickly or slowly you function).
- Trigger growth (as at puberty).
- Balance blood sugar.
- Affect the body's water balance.
- Regulate respiration (breathing).
- Determine cell metabolism (the rate at which cells function).
- Affect neural activity (the nervous system).

You can see what a varied and complex part hormones play in your life and how much they matter. One hormone cannot be viewed in isolation but rather must be seen as a component of a balance of circulating hormones.

A question of balance

Some women live their whole lives with no hormonal problems whatsoever. Periods come and go with minimum disruption, premenstrual syndrome (PMS) is unknown, there is little or no trouble before and after pregnancy. Even the contraceptive pill is swallowed without side-effects, and sterilization or hysterectomy produce no more than transitory difficulties.

But for other women, any interference with the hormonal system at any level causes chemical changes and alterations in body/mind rhythms, with resulting symptoms of hormonal distress.

Hormonal upset can arise from:
- The use of the birth control pill or other hormone-containing medicines.
- Hypothalamic or pituitary problems resulting from pregnancy, miscarriage, or abortion.
- Surgery such as tubal ligation (sterilization) or hysterectomy.
- Anorexia or bulimia.
- Trauma (e.g., as a victim of violence).

- Conditions such as ovarian cysts, polycystic ovaries, endometriosis, or uterine fibroids.

Changes in hormone levels can also occur if the immune system breaks down as a result of chemical poisoning or viral infection, since hormonal problems and immune system dysfunction are often linked. For example, the main problem may be hormonal imbalance, but this is exacerbated by an impaired immune system function causing chronic tiredness. Or the basic problem may be centered on the immune system, causing damage to the ovaries and thus affecting hormonal status.

Stress and lifestyle always play their part. For instance, female airline flight attendants often suffer menstrual instability because their biological "time clocks" are disrupted as they fly through different time zones. In dancers, the demand for lean, muscular bodies often leads to amenorrhea (an abnormal suppression or absence of menstruation). Traumatic experiences such as bereavement, divorce, and violence all destabilize hormonal equilibrium, as can loss of a job and moving to a new home or community.

Ovarian cysts An ovarian cyst is an abnormal, fluid-filled swelling that develops in the ovary. The most common type occurs when the egg-producing follicle of the ovary enlarges to produce a "follicular cyst." Cysts often produce no symptoms, but some cause acute pain or irregular bleeding.

Polycystic ovaries This condition is thought to occur because of an imbalance between luteinizing hormone and follicle-stimulating hormone produced by the pituitary gland. Multiple cysts develop in either one or both ovaries, and ovulation ceases.

Endometriosis This is a condition in which the cells that form the endometrium (lining of the uterus) develop outside their normal location, forming little clusters of tissue (called implants) outside the uterus.

Fibroids These are lumps of fibrous and muscular tissue found growing on all levels of the uterus, although they have also been discovered in other areas within the pelvis. They are known to shrink naturally in women as they near the menopause, but some researchers believe they are sensitive to estrogen and are more likely to grow when high levels of this hormone are present.

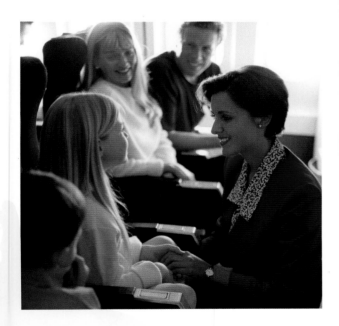

Frequent flying between different time zones can disrupt your biological "time clock".

The ovarian hormones

Of especial importance to women are the three hormones produced by the ovaries: estrogen, progesterone, and testosterone.

ESTROGEN

Estrogen is not really a single hormone. The word refers to a class of hormones that control female sexual development and promote the growth and function of female sex organs and secondary sexual characteristics. These estrogens include the hormones estradiol and estrone, which are essential for the health of the reproductive organs, and estriol, the predominant estrogen hormone during pregnancy.

Your body began producing estrogen when you were no more than a fetus, 15 to 20 weeks old, in your mother's womb. No doubt you have marvelled at the exquisitely soft skin of a baby. This is due to estrogen, which causes an extra layer of fat to develop and so makes the skin ultra soft.

At puberty, your level of estrogen increased dramatically, albeit erratically. Your breasts developed and the distribution of your body fat changed to produce the rounded contours of feminine hips and thighs. Maybe you can remember some of your emotions during puberty and adolescence—one day feeling elated and raring to go, the next apathetic and unhappy. These fluctuations are hardly surprising, given the bewildering and intricate changes that occur as your hormonal balance is established.

From this time, your life became influenced by the cyclic rise and fall in hormone levels involved in menstruation. For example, you may feel the stirrings of desire and the onset of sexual hunger in mid-cycle, at about the time your basal temperature readings indicate that you are at or near ovulation. This is the time at which both estrogen

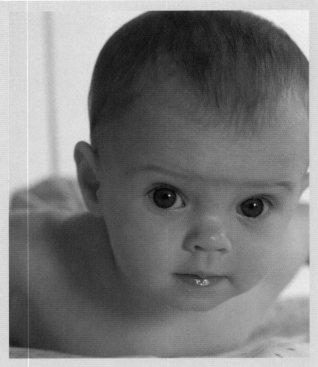

You can see how this baby's skin is beautifully soft and unblemished because of estrogen.

and progesterone levels peak, indicating a readiness for pregnancy.

Estrogen contributes to a healthy sex life, causing the vagina to moisten when aroused, and sensual areas to respond to stimulation.

As levels of estrogen decline during the menopausal years, the vaginal tissues become thinner and dryer. Estrogenic lubrication for sexual activity diminishes, and can result in vaginal penetration becoming uncomfortable and painful.

PROGESTERONE

Progesterone is produced primarily by the ovaries, although smaller amounts are also produced by the adrenal glands and large amounts by the placenta during pregnancy. Its role is to maintain the healthy functioning of the female reproductive system.

At the time of ovulation, the ovaries dramatically increase their output of progesterone, stimulating a woman's sex drive and preparing the lining of the uterus for fertilization. Adequate levels of progesterone are essential to the survival of the fertilized egg and the fetus. They are also thought to be responsible for the sense of well-being that is experienced by some women during their pregnancies.

Progesterone is known to be linked with mood and emotion. If you feel under par or even suffer premenstrual syndrome (PMS) at certain stages of your menstrual cycle, low levels of the hormone progesterone may be present.

It was the pioneering British gynecologist, Dr. Katherina Dalton, who pioneered the addition of progesterone for sufferers of PMS. She had terrible migraines with her menstrual cycle and discovered these could be alleviated by progesterone injections. Her discovery was strengthened by the fact that her migraines completely disappeared during the final months of pregnancy, which is when progesterone levels in the body soar. However, not all women in this situation respond the way she did.

Apart from its reproductive function, progesterone is needed for the production of other hormones, such as cortisol, which has an important role in the metabolism of carbohydrates, fats, and proteins and in the body's response to injury and infection.

The production of ovarian progesterone declines during the menopausal years as the reproductive process ends. But it is still very much involved throughout your body, as explained on page 62.

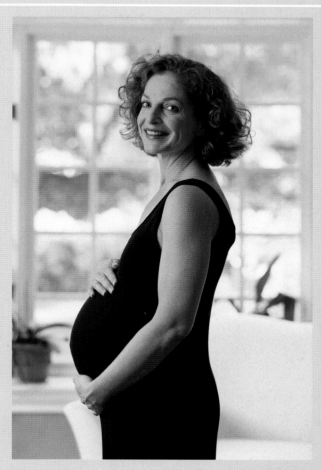

Hormonal balance contributes to the glow of healthy happiness seen in a pregnant woman.

PROGESTERONE CREAM

Nowadays, the most successful and most widely used type of progesterone preparation is transdermal progesterone (see page 65). This comes in the form of a cream and is applied to the skin. The progesterone is absorbed rapidly.

TESTOSTERONE

As well as being a major hormone for men, testosterone is also of great importance for women. Not only are the levels of testosterone in women's blood higher than the levels of estrogen, but their brains contain 20 times more testosterone than estrogen.

Men have 10 to 20 times more free testosterone than women. Half of a woman's testosterone is produced in the ovary and the other half in the adrenal gland. The hormone helps to determine secondary sexual characteristics, such as muscle mass and hair growth patterns, and adequate levels are essential for sexual desire, activity, and responsiveness in both men and women.

Nevertheless, while testosterone fuels the flames of desire, psychological factors determine the intensity and direction of the flame. The commonly held belief that hormones, in general, are the primary motivators of sexual activity in humans is a gross over-simplification. Hormones do not cause behavior; rather, they raise the likelihood that a given behavior will occur. Habit, circumstance, expectation, and conditioning can all have a more profound effect on behavior than hormones.

Testosterone levels decrease by about one-third in the average postmenopausal woman who still has her ovaries. If her ovaries are removed, the fall of testosterone is twice as great.

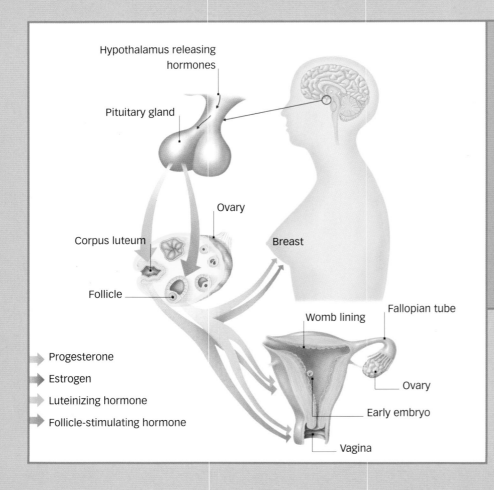

Hypothalamus releasing hormones

Pituitary gland

Corpus luteum

Ovary

Breast

Follicle

Progesterone

Estrogen

Luteinizing hormone

Follicle-stimulating hormone

Womb lining

Fallopian tube

Ovary

Early embryo

Vagina

THE HORMONE LOOP

Throughout the month, a constant feedback loop creates a continuous adjustment and regulation of the hormone levels between the hypothalamus and pituitary and the ovaries.

The change

The three hormones described earlier—estrogen, progesterone and testosterone—constantly change from day to day in a predictable and orderly rhythm. They determine when a woman is at her reproductive prime. This is a process with a beginning, a peak, a decline, and an end. Interestingly, humans are the only mammals in the world to experience this, all other female mammals reproduce until they die.

Central to a woman's reproductive life are her two ovaries. Estimates vary, but it is believed there are 6 to 7 million eggs present in a female fetus by the middle of its gestation. These begin to die off even before the child is born, but even so, the ovaries at birth contain somewhere between half-a-million and five million eggs. As the child develops, the eggs continue to die off; at puberty, 200,000 to 300,000 eggs remain.

Each time a woman ovulates, not one or two, but between 20 and 1,000 eggs are used up. Only one or two eggs per

During a woman's fertile years, one of her ovaries will ripen and release an egg once a month.

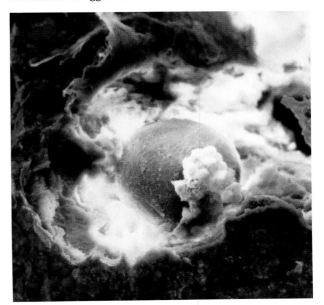

Perimenopause This is the period about two years before and two years after your final menstrual period. It is the time when you notice the most physical changes, such as irregular periods and hot flashes.

Menopause Your final menstrual period. Determining the date of your menopause can only be done retrospectively, after you have been free of menstruation for a full year.

Postmenopause These are the months and years that follow your final menstrual period. The postmenopause overlaps with the perimenopausal stage.

Climacteric This term comes from a Greek word meaning "rung of a ladder" and refers to the period of passage out of the reproductive stage of life and into the nonreproductive phase. It encompasses perimenopause, menopause, and early postmenopausal years.

cycle would have fully matured, and with increasing age, the eggs become used up more rapidly. Between the ages of 38 and 44, about 50,000 eggs are lost.

Ovulation slows down during the perimenopause. This is defined as the transition between the time you begin to experience menopausal symptoms (usually the mid to late 40s) and the time when your periods actually stop (average age of 51).

Many women find that they experience the menopause at the same age as their mothers did.

How do I know if I'm in my perimenopause?

The signs that herald the arrival of the perimenopause are varied. You might find yourself having two periods a month, and if you get a heavier flow, you may think you are always bleeding. Or you could go several months without bleeding. The actual flow may change, with lighter, more watery bleeding and less clotting because of reduced estrogen levels. The wide-ranging hormone-related symptoms of the perimenopause can be bothersome and include:

- Night sweats, interrupted sleep or insomnia.
- Irritability.
- Anxiety.
- Loss of concentration.
- Headaches (especially premenstrual migraines).
- Vaginal dryness.
- Vaginal atrophy (thinning of the vaginal walls due to lack of estrogen).
- Less interest in sex.
- Urinary stress incontinence.
- Mood swings.

Obviously, many of these symptoms are interconnected. For instance, if you have such severe night sweats that you develop insomnia, your concentration will suffer and you will be irritable.

Reverse puberty

Any mood swings may well strike a chord with your early adolescence, and indeed these hormonal changes are just like those at puberty. As mentioned earlier, an erratic production of estrogen played an essential part in your development at puberty. The fluctuating hormonal levels, coupled with the daily traumas of adolescent life, lead to the wild mood swings that are so much a part of being a pubescent girl.

In the perimenopause, the exact reverse happens but with similar results: the ovaries are winding down instead of gearing up, but the duelling hormonal levels can bring on the same mood swings you probably experienced all those years ago.

Is it me or is it hot today?

The most commonly experienced perimenopausal symptoms are hot flashes and night sweats. These occur in up to 25 percent of perimenopausal women and 50 to 85 percent of menopausal women. For most women, they happen over a period of one to two years, but as many as 25 percent of women have hot flashes for more than five years.

Hot flashes can cause considerable surprise and embarrassment. One moment you are busy working as usual, the next moment you suddenly feel a warm sensation rising up from your chest, spreading across your neck, up to your head and scalp. It's boiling hot in the room and beads of perspiration prickle your skin. After what seems an age, the heat is gone, you are wet with sweat, and almost immediately begin to feel chilled.

The sudden onset of a hot flash can be very unsettling, a feeling that continues until it has passed.

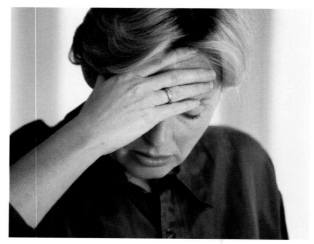

A typical hot flash lasts no more than three minutes, but it can range in duration from a few seconds to half an hour. It can be experienced in different ways. Some women have a specific focal point, such as the skin between the breasts, where the first tingles are felt, warning of an approaching hot flash. There may be no outward sign of redness or sweating—or you might sweat profusely and become as red as a beet. The sensation varies from mild discomfort to such intense feelings that you have to fight the urge to pull off your clothing.

At night, the flashes are called night sweats, and you may wake up to find yourself drenched in sweat, sometimes to the point where you need to get up, dry yourself, and change your night clothes. Women often complain that night sweats are worse than daytime flashes because:

- It is not possible to pick up the warning signals of an approaching flash while asleep, and do anything to lessen its impact.
- Disturbed sleep results in tiredness, depression, and irritability next day.

WHY DO HOT FLASHES HAPPEN?

The physiology of the hot flash is not yet fully understood, but the discomfort probably is caused by chemicals being released into the bloodstream at this time of hormonal disruption. The blood vessels are sensitive to the chemicals and dilate; blood then rushes to the skin, making you hot and red. A medical dictionary defines hot flashes as "vasomotor symptoms of the climacterium; sudden vasodilation with a sensation of heat, usually involving the face and neck, and upper part of the chest; sweats, often profuse, frequently follow the flash".

Hot flashes are termed "vasomotor" symptoms because the size of the blood vessels changes as part of the body's temperature-control system: blood vessels dilate (get larger) to allow more blood to move through to cool you down. Hot flashes are linked to the breakdown of

DID YOU KNOW?
Not all estrogen is lost when ovarian function ceases. The conversion of adrenal-gland hormones into estrogen (which had little importance before menopause) increases. This estrogen conversion occurs primarily in fat tissues. Because of this process, estrogen production continues for at least 10 to 20 years after menopause. This can be quite variable from woman to woman, which helps to explain why some women age more rapidly than others (an acceleration of skin aging is likely as estrogen levels decline.)

temperature control by the hypothalamus as estrogen production declines. They signal the end of your child-bearing years. This may be because:

- Your ovaries have used up all their eggs.
- Your ovaries no longer respond to the secretion of FSH from the pituitary as they once did by producing estrogen.

A few women go through the perimenopause overnight; periods will simply cease and these women have no associated symptoms. But most women experience some discomfort at this time and are aware of hormonal changes going on within their bodies that may or may not disrupt their lives. This is usually an erratic process: periods may come late or early, may be short, long, light, or heavy or may vanish for months and then suddenly reappear. It can take between two and five years to complete, and enormous changes take place in a woman's body as it acquires a new balance with lower levels of hormones.

The menopause is considered complete when periods have not occurred for one whole year.

Surgical removal of ovaries

For some women, the removal of the ovaries may be the only option if severe symptoms of pain, PMS, or endometriosis (see page 13) persist and all other treatments have been tried or if the ovaries are diseased.

Endometriosis is a disease affecting many women in their reproductive years, and it will recur as long as there is ovarian function. Although the ovaries themselves may be healthy, hysterectomy and removal of the ovaries is the only permanent cure. Endometriosis is the only disease that is "treated" by the surgical removal of tissue not directly affected by the disorder.

Some doctors advise against hormone replacement therapy for the first six months after surgery to remove ovaries. If all the endometrial implants are removed during the operation, the chance of a recurrence of the disease is slim. However, if even the tiniest deposit remains, then HRT will assist its growth.

All too often removal of ovaries is recommended for women aged 50 or older who are having a hysterectomy, the argument being that ovarian cancer may develop if they are retained. There is still considerable controversy about this issue, and if you are faced with this possibility, you need to weigh the risks of developing ovarian cancer against the benefits of continued ovarian function (i.e., hormone production). The latest research in the USA, Denmark, Japan, Australia, and the United Kingdom shows:

- Family risk factors include infertility, a well-documented family history of ovarian cancer, late menopause, and lack of child-bearing.
- Sterilization may reduce the risk of ovarian cancer by 39 percent.
- Hysterectomy may reduce the risk of ovarian cancer by 36 percent (although the Danish nationwide controlled follow-up study of ovarian cancer after hysterectomy [1997] suggests this protection might fade out with time).
- Women preserving at least one ovary have a significantly decreased risk of ovarian cancer for at least ten years after hysterectomy.
- Women who have heavy periods before hysterectomy tend to have a lower risk of ovarian cancer after surgery than women who have light or normal periods.

If you are still ovulating, then removing your ovaries will deprive you of significant hormonal support, which is difficult to replace adequately. The most critical issue is loss of bone mass leading to osteoporosis, which surgical removal of ovaries is known to initiate (see page 44). In menopausal years, the ovaries continue to secrete hormones that support your well-being and health.

PREMATURE MENOPAUSE

Whether you are 20 or 50 years old, surgical removal of ovaries is a very serious step to take (see also page 61). It leads to a premature menopause either immediately or within two years of the operation, and you are likely to be given a prescription for HRT. This may result in months of "trial and error" until the correct dosage is found to supplement your own reduced estrogen levels.

IMPORTANT

It is vitally important that you discuss all the issues and implications of HRT with your doctor if your ovaries are to be surgically removed.

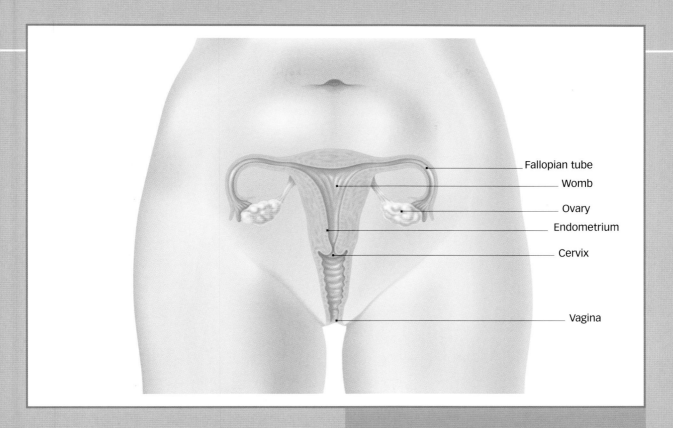

Fallopian tube

Womb

Ovary

Endometrium

Cervix

Vagina

THE REPRODUCTIVE SYSTEM

The main components of the reproductive system are the womb (uterus), fallopian tubes and ovaries. The outlet of the womb is the cervix which projects into the vagina.

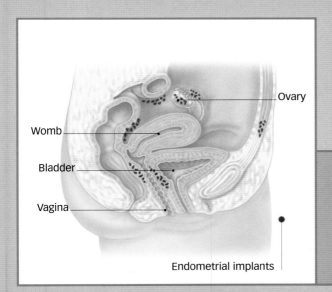

Ovary

Womb

Bladder

Vagina

Endometrial implants

ENDOMETRIOSIS

Here are some of the internal organs where deposits of endometriosis are commonly found.

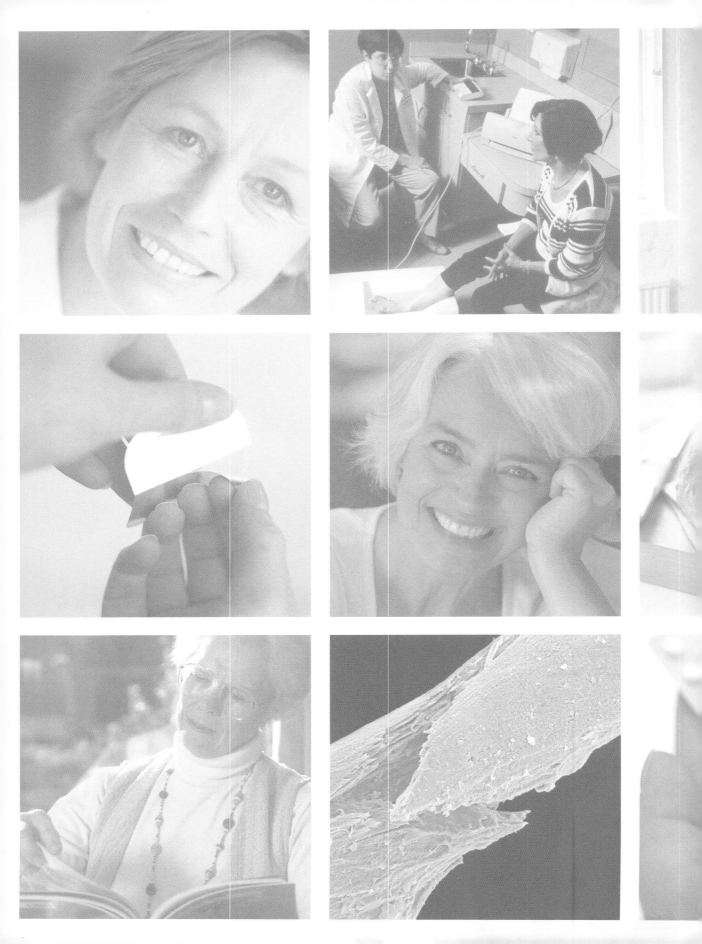

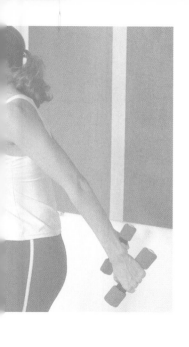

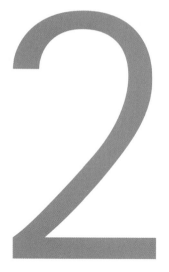

2

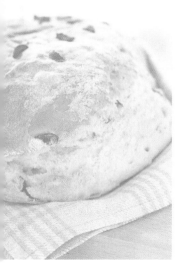

Hormone replacement therapy

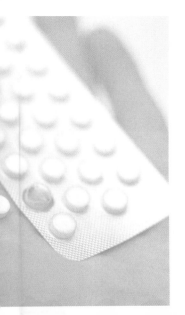

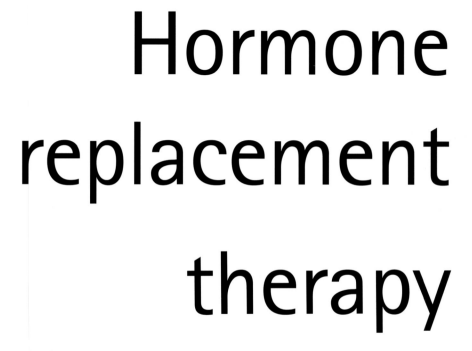

Considering hormone replacement therapy

Ever since early in the twentieth century, when the hormone estrogen was first found to be linked with the menopause, attempts have been made to use estrogen to alleviate menopausal symptoms. In the 1920s, extracts from the dried ovaries of sheep were used in early trials, and in the 1930s a "natural estrogen" extracted from the urine of pregnant mares was found to be effective.

By the mid-1960s estrogen therapy was hailed as "the pathway to eternal youth," promising to protect women from the "living decay" of their middle years. Wrinkly skin, middle-age spread, and sagging breasts would be eradicated, along with crying spells, violent mood swings, aching joints, and loss of memory. Replacing all this would be eternally feminine, sexually active menopausal women with glowing skin and glossy hair.

A driving force in the promotion of estrogen therapy at this time was a New York gynecologist, Dr. Robert Wilson, founder of the Wilson Foundation. The pharmaceutical industry generously contributed millions of dollars to the Foundation and funded aggressive promotional and advertising campaigns. Dr. Wilson's book, *Feminine Forever*, sold over 100,000 copies in its first year. Women's magazines eagerly seized upon his ideas, spreading the belief that the menopause was a kind of "living decay."

By feeding on women's greatest fears, Dr. Wilson struck a receptive chord. He extolled the virtues of estrogen replacement, which would save women from "the tragedy of menopause that often destroys their character

as well as their health." Fueled by a potent cocktail of vanity, anxiety, and media coverage, sales of estrogen rocketed, even though there had been no formal assessment as to its safety, let alone its long-term effects.

In the 1970s, however, panic set in when medical research showed that American women who took estrogen were 5 to 14 times more likely to develop cancer of the lining of the uterus (the endometrium) than those who were not taking estrogen. It appeared that the hormone stimulated growth of the endometrium and that this was leading to cancer in some cases. Understandably, the popularity of estrogen therapy waned.

New approaches were needed. One was the addition of progestogen (a synthetic form of the hormone progesterone) to the therapeutic regime. This "opposes" the action of the estrogen and allows the lining of the womb to be shed, as in a normal period, thus reducing the risk of cancer developing.

At this point the pharmaceutical industry abandoned its false claims that estrogen therapy preserved feminine

Lines and wrinkles are not something to be ashamed of—laughter lines reflect a contented life in middle years.

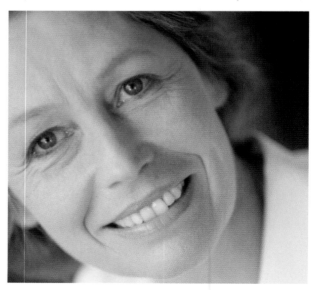

beauty and started to proclaim that the primary objective of the "new" hormone replacement therapy was the relief of menopausal symptoms.

So what exactly is HRT?

Hormone replacement therapy is an available treatment to replace or supplement a woman's estrogen levels when ovarian production decreases or stops during the menopause. As mentioned earlier, estrogen on its own provides no protection against the possibility of uterine cancer. The addition of a synthetic hormone, progestogen, provides that protection.

Although progestogens are able to fulfill many of the functions of progesterone, the human body has a certain degree of difficulty "recognizing" and coping with them. This is the cause of the well-known side-effects of mood swings and depression, which some women have when they start HRT.

The estrogen used in HRT comes in two basic forms: "synthetic" (produced in a laboratory from soy beans) and "natural" (extracted from pigs' ovaries or the urine of pregnant mares). The latter is used in the manufacture of two commonly prescribed preparations called Premarin and Prempak C. If you are concerned about animal welfare, you may not be too happy about taking an HRT preparation produced in this way.

In many ways the hormones used in HRT are exactly the same as the ones used in the contraceptive pill. The differences lie in the source of the estrogen and the dose. HRT uses either synthetic estrogen or "natural" estrogen extracted from pigs' ovaries or pregnant mares' urine, whereas the contraceptive pill contains the synthetic form of estrogen called ethinyl estradiol. The dose of estrogen is also much lower in HRT preparations.

The progestogens used in the contraceptive pill and HRT

are the same. The difference lies in the schedule: in HRT, they are given for only 10 to 12 days of each menstrual cycle.

Why should I consider taking HRT?

First, HRT is one option for you if symptoms of your climacteric are disrupting your physical and emotional well-being. You can assess the severity or otherwise of these by completing the chart on page 26.

Second, HRT is believed to provide protection from the possibility of cardiovascular disease or osteoporosis as you age, particularly if you are at risk from either condition for genetic or other reasons. In recent years, promising evidence has also emerged that it may offer protection against Alzheimer's disease (see pages 41–42) and bowel cancer (see pages 42–43).

DID YOU KNOW?

For six months of their pregnancies, an estimated 75,000 mares are confined in stalls on farms in Canada and the USA. These stalls are so small that the mares are unable to take a step or two in any direction. A harness is tied to the animal's rear quarters from which is attached a cumbersome urine-collection bag. This chafes their legs and prevents them from lying down comfortably. Outside exercise is occasional, if at all, and mares are given limited drinking water so that their urine will yield more concentrated estrogens. Some of the foals born are used to replace their exhausted mothers, many of whom have been confined on these farms for up to 20 years. But most are sold, fattened, and slaughtered for pet food.

MENOPAUSAL SYMPTOM CHART

Mark the box that most closely reflects how severely you are experiencing each of these symptoms.
Each box you marked has a score beside it.

Symptoms	Severe	Moderate	Mild	None
Hot flashes	12☐	8☐	4☐	0☐
Sweating attacks	12☐	8☐	4☐	0☐
Tension/irritability	3☐	2☐	1☐	0☐
Dryness of vagina/irritation	3☐	2☐	1☐	0☐
Loss of interest in sexual intimacy (ignore if not applicable)	3☐	2☐	1☐	0☐
Insomnia	3☐	2☐	1☐	0☐
Lack of energy	3☐	2☐	1☐	0☐
Hair/skin changes	3☐	2☐	1☐	0☐
Muscular and/or joint pains	3☐	2☐	1☐	0☐
Changes in memory/concentration	3☐	2☐	1☐	0☐

Once you have marked a box for each symptom, add up your score. A score of 30 or more strongly suggests
that symptoms are associated with the menopause, although a low score will not exclude this.

Will the doctor do any tests before prescribing HRT?

Your doctor should examine you thoroughly, especially your breasts and pelvis, and check your blood pressure. There are a few medical reasons for not using HRT, and it may not be suitable if you have a history of any of the following conditions:

- Endometriosis (unless it has been treated or has become quiescent postmenopausally)
- Breast cancer or cysts
- Cancer of the lining of the womb (the endometrium)
- Liver disease
- High blood pressure or stroke
- A personal and/or family history of clotting of the deep leg veins or the lungs
- Any estrogen-dependent malignancy
- Untreated vaginal bleeding

It is unlikely that you will be required to take a blood test, even though some women manufacture more estrogen than others, and the dose of HRT should be individualized according to hormone levels. For the most part, blood tests to accurately measure the levels of hormones in your body are useless and extremely unreliable.

The tests are only able to measure 1 to 9 percent of the biologically active hormones circulating in your body. There is now a better way. In recent years, the World Health Organization has been using saliva samples for an accurate reading of hormone levels.

When your salivary gland makes saliva it also secretes the biologically active forms of cortisone, testosterone, estrogen, and progesterone. This makes it possible to measure the levels of these hormones in a saliva test.

The Female Hormone Kit test, for example, is a very

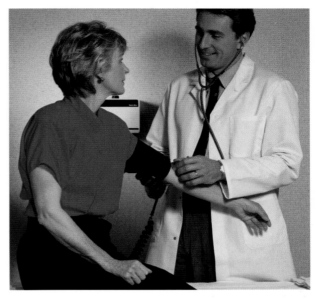

Your blood pressure should be monitored regularly by your doctor if you take HRT.

simple one which can be done in the privacy of your home with the samples you collect being sent for analysis. A total of 11 saliva samples are collected at specific times, and levels of estrogen, progesterone and testosterone are mapped to provide an accurate picture of your "hormonal highways." An interpretation of the test is provided when the results are returned. If you decide to have this test, you could discuss the findings with your doctor during the initial discussion about taking HRT.

> *I had awful night sweats, and within days of going on HRT I felt like a different person. I had so much more energy. I hadn't realized I was so tired because I think it tends to build up gradually and you get used to it.*
>
> *It's also helped me cope with work and my family better, especially as my husband and I are now managing a country hotel. I'm sure I couldn't work such long hours without HRT.*
>
> LYNN

Benefits and side-effects

What are the benefits of HRT for menopausal symptoms?

As soon as you start taking HRT, you are likely to find an improvement in the frequency and severity of hot flashes and night sweats, maybe within a week. This often leads to improved sleeping patterns and less daytime irritability, mood swings, etc. Women often report a general improvement in their energy levels, their ability to cope with the unexpected, and in their overall outlook and self-confidence. The full effect should be apparent by 12 weeks, when you should have your first critical review.

Relief from menopausal symptoms can transform your life.

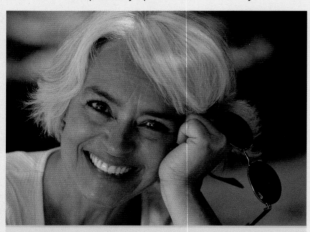

IS HRT THE ANSWER TO ALL SYMPTOMS?

HRT can be a useful diagnostic tool in eliminating symptoms that are estrogen-dependent. For instance, you might find that HRT has abolished your mood swings and irritability, yet you remain significantly depressed. If that happens, additional help, such as counselling, might be suggested by your doctor.

What about side-effects?

HRT causes "start-up" effects. These are the consequence of your body reacting to the presence once again of normal, adult levels of estradiol in your blood, sometimes after an absence of many years. You are highly likely to experience some, or all, of the following:

- Breast tenderness
- Nipple sensitivity
- Headaches
- Increase in appetite
- Calf muscle cramps

Infrequent or rare reactions include:

- Diarrhea
- Gastrointestinal upsets
- Muscular or joint pains
- Scalp hair loss
- Increased blood pressure
- Sensitivity to light
- Vaginal bleeding
- Breathing disorders
- Depression
- Acne
- Pains or swelling in upper leg
- Skin rash
- Heart palpitations
- Swollen ankles
- Migraines

If you experience any of these, you should see your doctor and discuss the situation, rather than waiting for your scheduled check-up.

HRT and weight gain

You may have friends or family who have gained weight when taking HRT, and you are concerned that it will happen to you.

In midlife, women tend to gain weight whether menopausal or not. However, after the menopause, this extra weight is distributed more in the abdomen than in the thighs and hips. Hormone replacement therapy effectively prevents the redistribution of body fat but does not prevent the weight gain itself.

Logic dictates that a gain in weight is inevitable if you take estrogen which turns the food energy into body fat. It is no coincidence that cattle are fed estrogen hormone to fatten them up for market. A sudden increase in weight is a common complaint after starting HRT, and the reason weight continues to rise is likely to be a combination of HRT, overeating, and inadequate physical exercise.

Research has shown that women on HRT do gain weight. Reality tells a different story, as borne out by anecdotal evidence.

If weight gain is an issue for you, prepare a diet diary if you are considering HRT or are on HRT. Take a separate page for each day of the week and on each one, line up columns with the following headings:

- Time you ate
- What food you consumed
- How much you ate
- What you were doing when you ate
- Where you ate
- With whom you ate, or if alone
- How you felt when you ate

Keeping this record will make you far more aware of what you really eat, and the psychological stimuli associated with your food intake. You might be surprised by what is revealed. For example, many people find that they "snack" much more than they realized or that they eat more if they are alone.

Make a note of your weight on day 1 of starting HRT. Record your diet diary (honestly!) for two weeks, and if you have put on weight, take immediate action. Discontinue the HRT for two weeks and monitor your weight. If it stays the same, modify your food intake and increase your physical exercise. Then continue the HRT for two weeks while continuing to modify your food intake and increase your physical exercise.

If you continue to gain weight in spite of making lifestyle changes, then you may need to discontinue the HRT and seek other solutions for your menopausal difficulties.

> I had a hysterectomy and ovariectomy when I was 30 years old because of endometriosis. Severe hot flashes and sweats started during the first two to four weeks after surgery, and I gained about 60 to 70 pounds (27 to 32 kilos) during the year I was on HRT. At first I used patches, but the glue caused a severe rash, so I went onto estrogen-only tablets. I decided to stop taking it and see how I felt. After several months, I went to the doctor and told him my menopausal symptoms had gone, so he agreed it was all right not to take HRT but that I would need regular bone scans.
>
> I lost about 20 pounds (9 kilos) in weight after stopping HRT and starting a healthier eating lifestyle. I don't agree with so much emphasis on raw foods, but I now eat more fruit and vegetables and have cut down on salt and fried foods.
>
> **STEPHANIE**

What types of HRT are available?

HRT preparations come in various forms. The main choices available at the present time, all of which contain various dosages of hormones, are tablets, patches, implants, vaginal creams, and rings.

TABLETS

This is the most common form of HRT, and there are more than 50 different tablets available. For women who have not had a hysterectomy (i.e., who have an intact uterus), tablets containing both estrogen and progestogen are usually prescribed. Sometimes the two hormones are combined in one tablet, sometimes they are taken separately in one of the following ways:

- **Cyclical therapy** Estrogen is taken for the first 21 days of the cycle; progestogen is taken from day 9 to day 21. Thus from day 21 there are seven days with no medication. Two days after the tablets are stopped, the fall in artificial hormone levels induces the womb lining to be shed, resulting in withdrawal bleeding. Such bleeds are not true periods but should resemble them in being less than a week in duration, not unusually heavy, relatively pain-free, and on time.
- **Continuous therapy** Estrogen is taken continuously every day and progestogen is taken from day 14 to day 25 of the menstrual cycle. Once the progestogen is finished, a withdrawal bleed occurs in the same way as in cyclical therapy. Continuous therapy is only prescribed for women over 54 years old or who have been without a period for one year.

Advantages of tablets
- Convenience. The pills are easy to take, neat, and easy to pack when traveling.
- It is easy to alter the dosage level, if necessary.

Disadvantages of tablets
- Irritation of a monthly bleed, especially if you thought your menopause meant freedom from menstruation.
- Some spotting and occasional bleeding is not unusual in the first six months of continuous therapy, and therefore many women prefer the predictability of the cyclic method. However, if you are willing to persist with continuous therapy, most women manage to overcome withdrawal bleeding and totally eliminate all periods within a year.
- Cost. In some health systems, patients find they need to pay for the two hormone tablets separately.

It is easy to keep track of HRT tablets as the daily dosage is prescribed in blister packs.

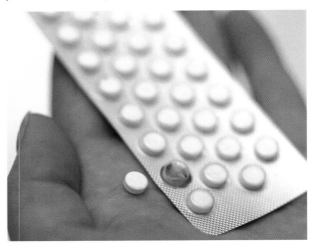

DID YOU KNOW?
If you have had a hysterectomy, you will not need progestogen because you no longer run the risk of endometrial cancer. Therefore, tablets containing only estrogen will be prescribed.

TIBOLONE (LIVIAL)

The synthetic steroid tibolone has the properties of estrogen, progestogen and androgen. One tablet per day is effective in reducing the severity and frequency of hot flashes and relieving sweating and headaches in postmenopausal women who have an intact uterus. It is not recommended for use until one year after the cessation of menstruation, since vaginal bleeding may occur in women who still produce their own estrogen.

Advantages of tibolone
- It is given as continuous therapy.
- It is helpful for women who cannot tolerate progestogens and the withdrawal bleeds associated with them.
- It has androgenic properties that are useful for maintaining libido and energy.

Disadvantage of tibolone
- It offers no advantage for women who have undergone a hysterectomy, either with or without oophorectomy (removal of ovaries).

TRANSDERMAL PATCHES

Transdermal estrogen patches contain tiny doses of estrogen that are released through the skin. You apply the patch to a small area on your buttocks or below your waistline, where the movement of your body will not cause the skin to wrinkle. The patch needs to be replaced every three to four days using a different site on your body. Progestogen is taken in pill form from days 14 to 25.

UNLUCKY FOR SOME
It is not unusual for women to get menopausal symptoms for many years after their periods stop. One study of Swedish women found that about 15 percent of them were still getting hot flashes 16 years after their last period.

There is a combined estrogen and progestogen patch available for women who still have a uterus. Again, the patch needs to be replaced twice weekly using a different site for the replacement.

Advantages of patches
- There is a gradual, constant absorption of hormone(s) into the bloodstream.
- The patch bypasses the liver, so this is a good alternative for women with a history of liver disease.
- No need to remember to take a pill every day.

Disadvantages of patches
- Some women have an allergic reaction to the adhesive, which can cause an itchy rash.

Transdermal patches are transparent and may wrinkle slightly when placed on the buttocks or waist.

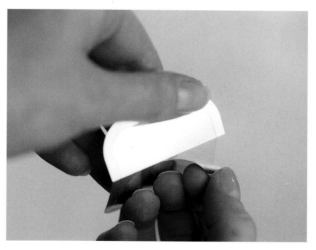

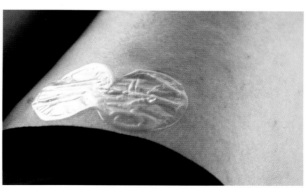

- You may initially become fidgety and hyperactive.
- The patch adheres well enough in the shower or when swimming but may not stay on for prolonged soaks in baths.
- Sweat can also unstick a patch: women who live in hot, humid climates and athletes who perspire heavily often report the patches becomes loosened more readily.
- Occasionally, a woman's partner may complain about the aesthetics of the patch, which is generally placed on the hip, thigh, or tummy. If this is a continuing problem, you might want to change to another form of HRT.
- You need to take progestogen tablets unless it is a combined patch.
- Cost. Patches are generally more expensive than tablets and you may need to pay separately for both the patches and the progestogen tablets.

> I was started on HRT in the form of tablets. These produced high blood pressure and headaches so I was changed to patches. They changed my life. The night sweats and flashes disappeared, as did the pain in my vagina.
> ANNETTE

A STICKY SUBJECT

Some women find that their patches don't stick to them very well. If this is a problem for you then try one of these methods for making your patch stay in place. Make sure that your skin is completely dry and free of all lotions, powders and oils before you apply on the patch. Alternatively, clean the area with alcohol and then blow dry with a hair dryer.

HORMONE IMPLANTS

Implants are little pellets that are inserted under the skin in a simple surgical procedure, either at a local surgery or in a hospital outpatient department. The doctor injects a little local anesthetic into the skin of the abdomen, a tiny cut is made in the skin, and an estrogen pellet (about the size of an apple seed) is inserted through a tube. The tube is removed, and the pellet is pushed down into the fat under the skin. The opening is closed either with a stitch or an adhesive strip.

The hormones are absorbed slowly from the pellet, and a single implant can last up to nine months, depending on the dose. For women who still have a uterus, the implant is combined with progestogen tablets.

Advantages of implants
- The estrogen bypasses your liver and goes straight into the bloodstream.

The insertion of an implant in the abdomen is a quick and painless procedure.

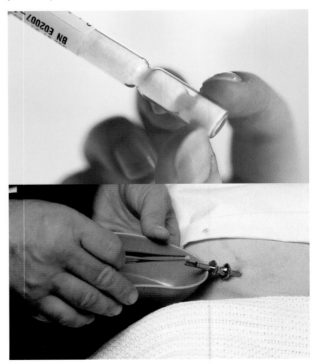

- Convenience. Once inserted, the implant can be forgotten. Return of menopausal symptoms signals the need for replacement of the implant.

Disadvantages of implants
- Once inserted, the implant cannot easily be retrieved; you have to wait until it has run its course if the dosage is incorrect.
- Unless you have had a hysterectomy, you need to take progestogen tablets to induce a bleed.
- The symptoms associated with the menopause appear to reoccur at shorter and shorter intervals, so that the implant has to be replaced more often.

NASAL SPRAYS

A relatively new development is a once-daily nasal spray that administers estrogen through a metered-dose pump. The hormone is absorbed through the lining of the nose and is said to mimic the way the natural hormone works. Women who have not had a hysterectomy still need to take progestogen for at least 12 days when using this type of HRT. Nasal sprays may not be appropriate for people who have persistent nasal problems, but can still be used if you just have a cold. At the publishing date of this book, estrogen nasal sprays are not available for use in the United States as they have not been approved by the USDA. They are being used extensively in several European countries, however, so this information may be of interest to you in the future.

Advantages of nasal sprays
- The estrogen is rapidly absorbed into the bloodstream and bypasses the liver and intestines.
- The spray relieves moderate to severe symptoms in both menopausal and postmenopausal women.
- Any change in dosage can be provided by adjusting the number of sprays.
- Cost is comparable to patches or gel.

Disadvantages of nasal sprays
- Long-term adverse effects or benefits have yet to be explored.
- Specifically, the effect on bone mineral density is still being evaluated.

VAGINAL CREAMS

After or during the menopause many women find that vaginal dryness makes sexual intercourse less enjoyable—or even painful. This happens because of insufficient estrogen. As we discussed earlier, the estrogen hormones are responsible for maintaining the shape, size, flexibility, and lubrication of the vagina. They hasten the flow of blood to the pelvic area during sexual arousal, and blood surges through the tissues, causing the release of fluid into the vaginal passage. This increased blood flow also makes the skin, nipples, and other sensual areas respond more pleasurably to stimulation, increasing sexual response and the quality of a woman's orgasm.

If estrogen is in short supply, vaginal tissues become dry and less pliable. The entrance to the vagina may become so narrow that intercourse is impossible. This effect may become more obvious if your adrenal glands have been depleted by stress, and you may be aware of gradual changes as estrogen levels diminish during the menopausal years.

TRIAL RESULTS
A six-nation trial of estrodiol nasal spray in 1999 showed symptoms were significantly reduced within four weeks, and 85 percent of women who took part in the trials elected to continue with this novel form of treatment. Tests showed that the effectiveness of nasal sprays was equal to that of tablets.

If sexual intimacy is part of your life, either with a partner or through masturbation, vaginal dryness can be treated with cream inserted directly into the vagina using an applicator-dose. Even if you are taking HRT in the oral or patch form, it may be necessary to use an estrogen cream to relubricate the vagina.

Advantages of vaginal creams
• Quickest way to treat vaginal dryness
• Easily reversible

Disadvantages of vaginal creams
• Creams can be messy.
• It is hard to control the dosage (taking too much estrogen can lead to overgrowth of the endometrium and the risk of developing endometrial cancer).
• The dose is too low to help with hot flashes.
• Creams should not be used directly before sexual intercourse with a man, unless he uses a condom, as he could absorb enough estrogen through his penis over time to cause him side-effects such as breast enlargement.

VAGINAL RINGS (ESTRING)

With this form of HRT, a vaginal ring made of silicon is inserted high into the vagina, where it stays for three months. During this time, the ring releases a low dose of estrogen locally. Replacements can be inserted at three-month intervals for a period of up to two years. The ring provides a very low dosage of estrogen only to the vagina, so many doctors believe it is safe to use vaginal rings to treat vaginal dryness or atrophy in women who have had breast cancer. Neither the woman nor her partner can feel the ring during intercourse, but if you or your partner find the ring uncomfortable or unacceptable, it can be removed and replaced afterwards.

Advantages of a vaginal ring
• It can be removed easily if a problem develops.
• Estrogen levels remain constant as long as the ring is in place.

Disadvantages of a vaginal ring
• Some women dislike the idea of "something up there."
• Women who have had a hysterectomy may have trouble keeping the ring in place, especially if the vagina has been shortened in the operation.

An applicator may not have the flexibility of a tampon, but it is just as simple to insert in a vagina.

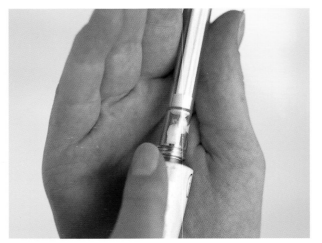

Vaginal rings are flexible and easy to handle. They are inserted high into the vagina and release a very low dose of estrogen.

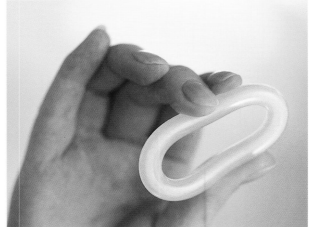

HRT and breast cancer

CLINICAL TRIALS

Clinical trials/studies are generally of four types:

- A *Prospective study* can be placebo-controlled (where half the participants receive dummy pills), double-blinded (where neither experimenters nor the participants know the particulars of the test items), single-blinded (where the experimenters but not the participants know the particulars of the test items), or unblinded (where both experimenters and participants know the particulars of the test items).
- A *Retrospective study* looks back after the effect has happened. For example, when people develop a condition, researchers look back to discover whether any particular factor contributed to it.
- A *Case-control study* is helpful in finding out the correlation between A and B factors in a rare medical condition.
- An *Observational study* can be helpful in finding out a correlation between two apparently unrelated factors. A good example of this is when it was found that many people working in an asbestos factory developed lung cancer.

In addition, researchers sometimes use *meta-analysis*. This is where similar prospective studies are pulled together and all of them are analyzed as a single study. This often reveals a better picture of the medical situation.

Considerable contention and uncertainty about HRT relates to the risk of breast cancer—a disease that affected over a million people worldwide in the year 2000, one-third of whom live in Europe. The uncertainty is not helped by conflicting studies, some of which show the risk of breast cancer is reduced by HRT while others suggest a slight increase.

This controversy is clearly illustrated by the publication in the journal *The Lancet* (1997) of a report that re-analyzed the raw data of over 90 percent of the worldwide studies of HRT and breast cancer. Individual data on nearly 53,000 women with breast cancer and just over 100,000 women without breast cancer from 51 studies in 21 countries were collected, checked and analyzed. The report concluded that:

> *"The risk of having breast cancer is increased in women using HRT and increases with increased duration of use. This effect is reduced after cessation of use of HRT and has largely, if not wholly, disappeared after about 5 years."*

Reading this, you might justifiably assume that the issue is now cut and dried. Not so. Many of the studies in this report were of women who had taken estrogen-only HRT, whereas most women these days use combined estrogen and progestogen HRT. The breast cancers in women taking HRT were found to be smaller, more compact, and less advanced than those found in women who were not taking HRT. However, that may be scant consolation for women and their families suffering the trauma of diagnosis, treatment, and potential recurrence of the cancer.

Three years later, researchers at the National Cancer Institute in Rockville, Maryland, released the results of a study of just under 45,000 postmenopausal women who took part in a breast cancer detection project between 1980 and 1995. The findings confirmed the potential hazards and uncertainties in the use of HRT and showed that:

- The relative risk of developing breast cancer was 20 percent higher for women who had taken HRT containing estrogen than for women who had never taken HRT.
- The risk was 40 percent higher for women who had taken estrogen with progestogen.
- Thin women were more at risk if they took estrogen alone.

More recent confirmation of this risk was made in 2002 when a US trial to evaluate estrogen and progestogen use in 16,000 postmenopausal women was stopped early by the Women's Health Initiative because health risks exceeded health benefits by a small margin.

Although the number was small, women receiving this particular HRT—Prempro (a continuous combined HRT tablet marketed only in the USA)—had a higher rate of breast cancer and more adverse cardiovascular events (i.e., coronary heart disease and stroke) than those receiving placebo, although there were benefits for hip fractures and bowel cancer. As the average age of the women was 63 years, it is hardly surprising there were no significant cardiovascular improvements. The degenerative effects of aging were already apparent, and the ground that had been lost could not be reclaimed.

It is no surprise to find that doctors are divided about the possible links between breast cancer and HRT when faced with such complicated findings: Some of them regard the risk of breast cancer as a very small one indeed; others believe the risks are unacceptable. A baffled response to a leading article on the subject in the British Medical Journal (December 2001) summed up one doctor's desperate plea:

SELF-EXAMINATION
It is important to know how to check your breasts yourself.

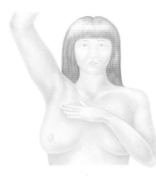

Check each breast for lumps, differences in skin texture and changes around the nipple. Feel right into each armpit.

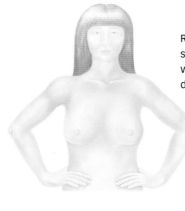

Repeat this check in several positions and with your arms in different postures.

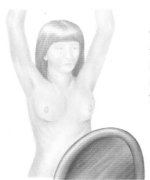

Try standing in front of a mirror to help you become more familiar with your breasts.

How is the typical working GP (or hospital clinician) to interpret supposedly "authoritative" advice when it is so emphatically contradicted by others apparently equally well-qualified?

THE WAY FORWARD FOR YOU

Before you can make an informed decision about whether to take HRT or not, you need to understand the risks as they apply to *you* and no other woman. It is certainly true that:

- Breast cancer happens whether women are taking HRT or not taking HRT.
- Breast tissue is influenced by changing levels of hormones.
- Other factors that determine the development of cancers include heredity and alcohol consumption.
- Some types of breast cancer are fast-growing and quickly fatal.
- Others develop very slowly, over 18 to 20 years or even longer.

It is important to consider all the risk factors that apply to you. Two possible areas related to breast cancer currently under investigation are (1) estrogen-containing preparations, such as the contraceptive pill and HRT, and (2) dietary factors.

Breast cancer and estrogen

Both the contraceptive pill and HRT contain estrogen, and it is known that estrogen can stimulate cancer cells to grow. In theory, increasing the supply of estrogen could trigger a breast cancer to develop; in practice, the risk of this happening appears to be a small one. Recent research looking at the contraceptive pill worldwide has revealed that:

- The incidence of breast cancer is increased slightly while the pill is taken and for up to 10 years after stopping.
- More than 10 years after stopping, the risk is the same as that of a woman who has never taken the pill.
- A large number of women diagnosed with breast cancer have used the contraceptive pill during the progression of their malignant disease process.

Breast cancer and diet

So far, the search for dietary factors implicated in breast cancer during adulthood has been disappointing. This does not preclude a possible association between breast cancer and diet *earlier* in life. The only fairly well-established dietary risk for breast cancer is alcohol; a small but consistent increase in risk has been associated with alcohol consumption.

Regular mammograms offer reassurance to women as potentially cancerous changes can be detected early.

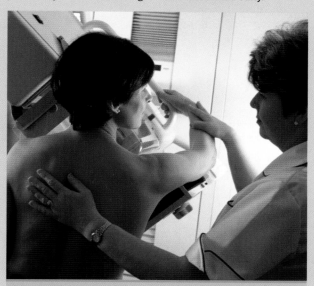

CHECK IT OUT

More than a million women who attended breast screening centers in the United Kingdom have volunteered to take part in "The Million Women Study," one of the most ambitious studies of women's health ever undertaken. It aims to answer questions about links between HRT and breast cancer and heart disease. The impact of HRT and other lifestyle factors on heart disease, bone disease, and joint replacement are also being investigated, as are diet, reproductive history, vitamin and mineral use, and family history of illness.

How long can I use HRT for menopausal symptoms?

How long you continue to use HRT will depend on your symptom relief. Some women decide to take it for six months, then discontinue it for a few months and see what difference this makes to their well-being. The symptoms may return during this time, because HRT often just "damps" them down, especially if they are severe. In this case, you might decide to:

- Restart the therapy.
- Change your method of HRT, e.g., from tablets to patches.
- Explore other solutions for your particular circumstances.

How do I get off HRT for good?

Before you stop taking HRT, seek the advice of your doctor. If you stop taking the medication abruptly, you may experience symptoms of rapidly falling levels of estrogen, such as hot flashes, migraines, and vaginal dryness. These symptoms are a form of withdrawal, and it is not advisable to go "cold turkey." In most cases, the recommended guidelines for coming off HRT are to do it gradually over three months. For the first month, substitute natural progesterone cream as described on pages 65–66 for the progestogen and reduce the estrogen by 50 percent. In the second month, reduce the estrogen by 50 percent again, and again for the third month. By the end of this month, the HRT can be safely and completely discontinued. You need to continue using the natural progesterone for the next three months.

You may find the use of natural progesterone leads to an experience of high estrogen effects—fluid retention, tenderness and swelling of the breasts, or even the appearance of scant vaginal bleeding. These effects are only temporary and will normally soon clear.

What about taking HRT postmenopausally?

Some doctors are cautious and believe that all HRT should be discontinued by 10 years after periods have ceased, mainly because of the greater risk of breast cancer in women from their 60s onward. Certainly, its continuing use after the age of 60 should be critically reviewed every five years. Having said that, it is not unknown for much older women to be taking HRT.

I am 84 years old and have been taking HRT for 30 years with no side-effects whatsoever. I have felt so fit and well, especially sexually. I have had three very happy relationships since my husband died 12 years ago, the last with a gentleman of 92.

My doctor recently refused to prescribe HRT again because of the recent findings about the increase in blood clotting when sitting for such long hours in an airplane when I visit family in Australia. I was very unhappy about this, so I changed my doctor and am now back on HRT.

LIZ

Other known benefits of taking HRT

We have already looked at the benefits to be had by taking HRT for the alleviation of menopausal symptoms, and Liz has confirmed the "feel-good" factors of fitness and high energy postmenopausally. There are other possible long-term benefits as well. Many doctors regard HRT as an acceptable lifelong adjunct to continuing good health, especially for women at risk of any of the following: Alzheimer's disease (see pages 41–42), bowel cancer (see pages 42–43), osteoporosis (see pages 44–52) and cardiovascular disease (CVD) (see pages 53–59).

Alzheimer's disease

Alzheimer's disease (also called presenile dementia) was named after a German doctor, Alois Alzheimer (1864–1915). He published many papers on conditions and diseases of the brain, one of which involved memory loss, behavior and personality changes, as well as a decline in cognitive abilities.

These clinical definitions in no way convey the pain and heartbreak experienced if you are intimately involved with someone who develops the disease. The actual degenerative process begins in midlife and is almost impossible to reverse.

RISK FACTORS

You are at increased risk of Alzheimer's disease if you have high blood pressure and/or high levels of cholesterol (as outlined on page 53) or if one of your parents or grandparents had or has the disease.

One theory is that you may be at extra risk if you undergo a dramatic loss of estrogen at menopause, as evidenced by symptoms such as memory lapses and erratic concentration. Given that the hypothalamus at the base of the brain acts as a control center for your hormones, it would seem logical to assume that a major hormonal disturbance would be bound to have an effect on the brain.

REDUCING THE RISK

Women who take HRT report that their ability to remember things improves almost immediately. This may be attributed to estrogen's effect on the growth of nerve cells or improved blood flow to the brain. In addition, estrogen may affect neurotransmitters, such as serotonin.

Regardless of the HRT regimen, there may be a "critical window" in the early stages of Alzheimer's disease when HRT may prevent a progressive loss of mental faculties.

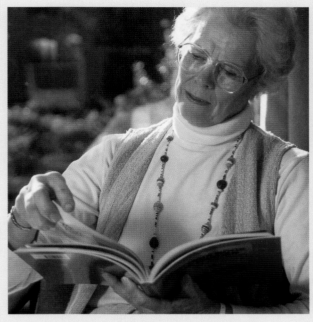

Some women continue to take HRT postmenopausally.

Dementia This is a deterioration of mental faculties combined with emotional disturbances resulting from an organic brain disorder. Alzheimer's disease is a degenerative disease of the brain that occurs in middle age and causes a progressive loss of mental faculties.

Serotonin An organic compound found in both animal and human tissue, especially the brain, blood, and the lining of the digestive tract. It is capable of raising body temperature and contracting smooth muscle and has a role in changing behavior and mood.

Neurotransmitters These are chemicals involved in the transmission of a nerve impulse between nerve cells.

Some experts believe that the prevention of Alzheimer's disease may become the primary reason for the prescription of HRT.

SUMMARY

- Neither dementia nor Alzheimer's disease are necessarily part of the aging process. It is therefore very important to consider the implications for you if your family medical history includes either of them, especially if you have high blood pressure and/or high levels of cholesterol.
- Current research indicates HRT is beneficial if you are at risk of both dementia and Alzheimer's disease.

HRT AND DEMENTIA

Researchers in the USA studied 1,124 elderly women with an average age of 74 years, who were assessed as nondemented. During follow-up, which ranged from 1 to 5 years, they discovered that:

- Of the 968 women who had never used HRT, 158 (16 percent) developed dementia.
- Of the 156 women who had taken HRT at the menopause, 9 (5 percent) developed the disorder.
- None of the 23 women who were taking HRT when the study started developed dementia.

Bowel cancer

Nearly a million people were diagnosed with bowel cancer worldwide in the year 2000. It is much more common in the Western world than in Asia and Africa, and it is believed to be due to differences in diet. Jewish people who are Ashkenazi or of Eastern European descent, are at increased risk of bowel cancer, and it is believed that a specific gene mutation can be found in 6 percent of this population.

Bowel cancer is the second leading cause of all-cancer death in the USA. It can occur at any age but is most common in the elderly and is rare in women under 40. The lifetime risk of developing it is about 1 in 20 for women. Nine out of ten cancers of the colon and rectum develop because of sporadic mutations in the cells lining the bowel. Sporadic mutations, which happen at random, accumulate over time and are caused by diet and the effects of advancing age.

RISK FACTORS

One of the risk factors is a family history of the disease. Certain criteria indicating a pattern of bowel cancer throughout generations can be evaluated using the Amsterdam Criteria. These state that a person's risk of developing bowel cancer is high if their family includes:

- At least three members with colon or rectal cancer.

THE PARADOX

The risk of bowel cancer in women before the menopause is doubled if they are clinically obese, although paradoxically, after the menopause the fat tissue is an important source of estrogen, which may reduce the risk of colorectal cancer.

- At least two successive generations with colon or rectal cancer.
- Two family members with the disease who are first-degree relatives (i.e., parents, brothers, sisters, or children) of another family member with colon and rectal cancer.
- At least one member affected at or before the age of 50.

Over the last 20 years, death rates from bowel cancer have dropped more in women than men, and accumulating evidence suggests that postmenopausal hormone use may decrease the risk of it.

In 1976, just under 60,000 postmenopausal registered nurses in 11 states in the USA took part in the Nurses Health Study, part of which examined the relationship between postmenopausal hormone therapy and bowel cancer. The follow-up lasted 14 years, and its findings showed a reduction in risk of 35 percent among women currently using postmenopausal hormones. However, the apparent reduction substantially diminished upon cessation of therapy. This study is one of 23 observational studies that suggest a 20 percent reduction in occurrence of bowel cancer in postmenopausal women who use HRT.

SUMMARY

- You need to consider the implications for you if your family medical history indicates you are at risk of this cancer.
- Improving and modifying your eating lifestyle will be of benefit.
- Considerable research indicates a marked reduction in occurrence of bowel cancer due to HRT.

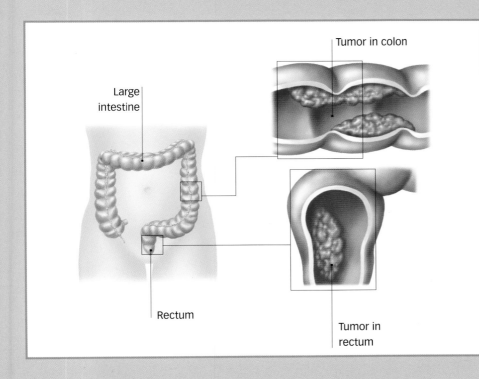

Tumor in colon

Large intestine

Rectum

Tumor in rectum

WHERE DOES BOWEL CANCER DEVELOP?
Bowel cancer usually affects the last part of the large intestine and the rectum.

Osteoporosis

The skeleton is a living organism that is continually renewing itself. Bone constantly undergoes breakdown and rebuilding in a controlled process necessary for bone growth and repair. This is known as remodeling.

The basic structure of bones does not change with age, but their density and strength will decrease. This is part of the natural aging process for men as well as women, but for some of us, bone is lost much faster than new bone can be formed to replace it. If this happens, bones can become so fragile that they are liable to break very easily; fractures commonly occur at the wrist, hip, and spine. Consequences can be devastating, and about 20 percent of patients who have hip fractures die.

This fractured bone has jagged edges. Consequently, it will take time for it to knit together.

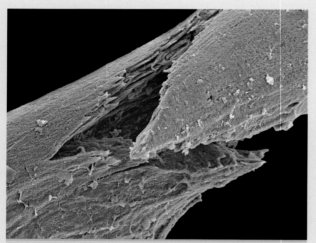

DID YOU KNOW?
Ten million Americans have osteoporosis; 80 percent of them are women. Each year the disease is responsible for 1.5 million fractures of the vertebrae, hip, wrist, and other bones.

The condition known as osteoporosis is a worldwide disease, as evidenced by the formation of support, information, and research organizations for osteoporosis in 70 countries. Racial origin influences a woman's risk of brittle bones. For example, women of African, Aboriginal, or Mediterranean extraction are unlikely to suffer osteoporosis because they usually have thicker bones and a greater bone mass at skeletal maturity. On the other hand Caucasian, Asian, or Oriental women generally have thinner bones and lower bone mass and therefore face a greater risk.

Osteoporosis can begin anywhere from 5 to 20 years before the menopause when estrogen levels are still high. It accelerates for a few years at the menopause or if the ovaries are surgically removed or nonfunctioning, as after a hysterectomy. At such times, the rate of bone loss increases from 2 to 5 percent a year. However, for some women the foundation for osteoporosis may well have been laid many years earlier by a diet grossly deficient in calcium or by a demanding athletic schedule that inhibited ovulation.

Osteoporosis is a silent disease that goes unnoticed and is usually painless in the early stages. Because you cannot see your bones, you may not know there is anything amiss until you break your hip, spine, or wrist after a minor bump or fall. Other symptoms include:

- Loss in height.
- A curving spine.
- Acute and unexplained back pain.

Osteoporosis can lead to a dramatic loss of height, severe curvature of the spine, chronic pain, and permanent disability. It can literally devastate lives, and the everyday activities that we all take for granted can become impossible.

RISK FACTORS

The following factors place you at high risk of osteoporosis:

- Very early menopause (before the age of 45), with early loss of estrogen as the ovaries stop working.
- Early menopause (before the normal age of 50), since early loss of estrogen is likely or certain if your ovaries are removed.
- Long-term use of high-dose corticosteroids (for conditions such as arthritis and asthma). Do not stop taking them; your doctor may be able to adjust your dosage to compensate for bone loss.
- Irregular or infrequent menstruation. This can happen naturally or be caused by over-exercising, anorexia nervosa, or bulimia. This results in low estrogen levels similar to menopause, regardless of age.
- Disorders of the digestion that cause malabsorption problems, such as celiac disease, Crohn's disease, or gastric surgery.
- Heavy smoking. This can damage bone-building cells and cause an early menopause.
- Low calcium intake. Consumption of calcium-rich foods helps maintain bone density.
- Heavy drinking. Alcohol abuse destroys bone.
- Immobility. Bones need exercise to remain strong, so those who are bed- and wheelchair-bound are more at risk.
- Lack of sunshine. Exposure to sunlight is necessary for vitamin D production, which is essential for bone health as a bone hardener.

Much of the variation in bone mineral mass and the incidence of osteoporosis can be ascribed to genetic differences. Therefore, a family history of osteoporosis puts you more at risk of having fractures later in life. If you are aware of a history of osteoporosis in your family, you should ask your physician about bone density testing.

> *I began suffering very strong back pain in 1995 and thought it was just the "aging" effect. But as time went on, my agility and mobility plummeted, and I had to depend more and more on my family for help. Visits to the doctor led to painkillers, then stronger painkillers, and I lost three precious years before I was found to have suffered severe loss of bone density.*

> CARMEN

DRINK MORE MILK

In 1994, a cross-sectional study of 284 women aged 44 to 74 living in Cambridge, UK, revealed that frequent milk consumption before the age of 25 was associated with 5 percent higher hip bone mineral density in middle-aged women and older women.

DID YOU KNOW?

A child's skeleton is replaced every two years, an adult's every 7 to 10 years. After bones have stopped growing in length at the age of 16 to 18 years, they still increase in density. After about age 35, they begin to deteriorate.

DIAGNOSIS

The best way to identify osteoporosis in its early form is by a test called dual energy X-ray absorptiometry (DXA), often referred to as a DXA scan. This can detect tiny amounts of bone loss of 1 to 3 percent, and regular yearly scans allow the rate of loss to be calculated.

At present, this method of bone density scanning is the most accurate and reliable method of assessing the strength of your bones. A DXA scan is usually done on your lower spine and one hip. Other areas that can also be assessed include your forearm and heel. Bone density is then compared with that of young, healthy adults.

DXA machines are expensive and may not be readily available. A less expensive diagnostic method uses a portable ultrasound machine that can assess bone structure and strength, usually of your heel bone (calcaneus), wrist, or finger. Heel ultrasound is also useful in predicting your osteoporotic fracture risk around the time of menopause and of Colles (wrist) fracture in your early postmenopausal years.

BONE DENSITY TESTING
Whatever is used to predict osteoporotic fractures, a measure of bone mass is only reliable when it is "read" (interpreted) by a medical doctor experienced in bone mass measurement.

REDUCE YOUR RISK BY INVESTING IN YOUR BONES

Your bones need calcium
Calcium accounts for about 67 percent of bone weight and bones act as a storage bank for calcium. If the amount of calcium in your blood falls below a certain level, your body will take its calcium needs from your bones. This calcium withdrawn from your bones is used for other important needs, such as those of the heart, muscles, blood, and nerve maintenance and repair.

Clearly, it is important to maintain your intake of dietary calcium. The chart opposite sets out ways in which you can increase this. However, it is also important to be aware of the way that other substances in foods and drinks can affect your calcium levels.

Substances that can reduce calcium absorption, when taken in large quantities, include:

- Phytates, present in fiber, particularly unprocessed bran.
- Tannins, present in tea.
- Oxalate, present in spinach.
- Caffeine, present in coffee, tea and cola drinks.
- Phosphates without calcium, found in fizzy, canned drinks.

Increasing your calcium intake

Daily requirement

before menopause 1,000 mg

after menopause 1,500 mg

Calcium content of common foods in milligrams per 100 g (approx 3½ oz) of food

DAIRY

Cheese	
Cheddar	800
Cottage	80
Danish blue	580
Edam	740
Parmesan	1,220
Processed	700
Spread	510
Cream	79
Egg (whole)	52
Egg (yolk)	130
Milk (1%)	
0.5 liter (1pint)	702
Milk (skim)	
0.5 liter (1pint)	705
Yogurt (low fat)	180
Ice cream	134

VEGETABLES

Beans, green	180
Beans, kidney	140
Broccoli	100
Cabbage	53
Chick peas	140
Greens, kale	98
Olives in brine	61
Parsley	330

Peas	31
Spinach	600
Spring onions	140
Watercress	220
Baked potato (large)	24
Baked beans	
(350 g/12¼ oz can)	239

MEAT AND FISH

Meat and fish contain very small amounts of calcium. Fish in batter contain calcium in the flour. Canned pilchards and sardines, salmon and whitebait contain calcium in the bones.

Prawns	150
Crab (canned)	120
Pilchards (canned)	300
Salmon (canned)	93
Sardines (canned)	460–550
Herring, sprats (fried)	620–710
Smelt, whitebait (fried)	860
Fish paste	280
Steamed scallops	120

FRUIT

Apricots, dried	92
Black currants	60
Currants	95
Figs	280
Lemon, whole	110
Rhubarb	100
Orange (1 large)	99

NUTS

Almonds	250
Brazil nuts	180
Peanuts, roasted and	
salted	61
Sesame seeds	870

DRINKS (DRY WEIGHT)

Cocoa powder	130
Coffee, ground	130
instant	160
Malted milk drink	230
Tea, Indian	430

FLOUR AND BAKED FOODS

Bread, white or brown	100
Cake, sponge	140
Flour, plain	210–40
self-raising	350
Soy flour	210–40
Wheat bran	110

COOKING INGREDIENTS

Curry powder	640
Mustard, dry	330
Pepper	130
Salt	230
Stock cubes	180
Yeast, dried	80

Substances that increase the loss of calcium in your urine include:

- Salt. A high salt intake increases urinary calcium loss.
- Protein. Excessive intake of protein from animal sources (more than four servings a day) lowers calcium levels.
- Caffeine. Coffee, tea and other caffeine-containing drinks increase output of urine, which promotes the loss of calcium.

Your bones need vitamin D

Vitamin D enhances calcium absorption. It is present in apples, watercress, tuna, salmon, and herring. But the best source of vitamin D is sunlight, which increases vitamin D production in the skin.

Your bones need magnesium

Magnesium is essential for the proper metabolism of calcium, and your bones need twice as much magnesium as calcium if the biochemistry of your bone formation is to run smoothly. Good sources are dark green vegetables, apples, seeds, nuts, figs, and lemons, as well as whole grains, such as brown rice, whole wheat, and whole rye.

Your bones need vitamins C, B6 and K

Vitamin C is crucial for bone formation because it produces collagen (fibrous matter), which makes up 90 percent of the bone matrix. Good sources of vitamin C include citrus fruits (oranges, lemons, limes), green and leafy vegetables, berries, potatoes, sweet potatoes, and yams.

Vitamin B6 appears to increase the strength of connective tissue in bones. It is found in wholegrains, fish, nuts, bananas, and avocados.

Vitamin K is known primarily for its effect on blood clotting, and it helps to harden bone. The best source is green vegetables.

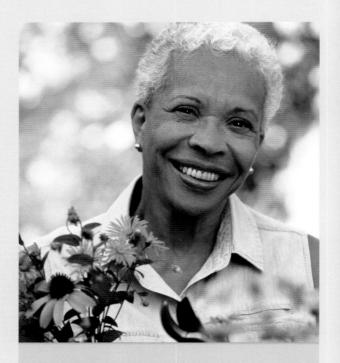

DID YOU KNOW?

Gardening boosts self-esteem, builds confidence, and may soon be prescribed by doctors.
Thrive (formerly the Society for Horticultural Therapy)

Your bones need exercise

The best type of exercise to strengthen bones is weight-bearing exercise. Your bones need to be loaded as you move. Good weight-bearing exercises include walking, jumping, ice-skating, running, skipping, ball sports, running up and down stairs, digging the garden, aerobics, and tennis. You should try to exercise for 20 minutes a day at least three times a week.

WHAT ELSE CAN BE DONE?

The good news is osteoporosis can be treated. If you are diagnosed with osteoporosis or have sustained fractures from the disease, you should be aware that it is never too late to begin treatment. There are a range of medications and treatments available that have been shown to be effective in slowing or halting bone loss and helping to prevent fractures. These treatments include the following options.

Bisphosphonates

This relatively new class of drugs is a nonhormonal type of treatment. Bisphosphonates allow bone-building cells to work more effectively, consequently resulting in increased bone density.

Three bisphosphonates currently available are:

- Risedronate (trade name Actonel), which has been shown to increase bone density and reduce the risk or frequency of fractures at the spine and hip.
- Alendronate (trade name Fosamax), which also increases bone density and reduces the frequency of fractures at the hip and spine.
- Etidronate (trade name Didronel), which also has been shown to increase bone density and reduce the risk of fracture in the spine but not the hip.

Selective estrogen receptor modulators (SERMs)

SERMs are a special class of drug with many features similar to estrogen in HRT. However, they differ in

FRACTURED BONES IN EUROPE

A European audit of osteoporotic fractures published in December 2001 disclosed the following rates per 10,000 people:

Sweden	20.1	Italy	13.6
Denmark	17.9	Greece	12.3
Germany	16.4	France	9.1
UK	14.4	Portugal	8.2

DID YOU KNOW?

Walking, running, aerobics classes, weight-lifting, dancing, and many other 'weight bearing' activities help build bone strength. However, too much of a good thing can be bad. The intense training of elite athletes and dancers can actually reduce bone density. Women who are training at this level need to be especially careful about their calcium intake and other nutritional support.

that they do not stimulate the breast and uterine tissues and, as a result, SERMs have the positive effect of estrogen on bone without increasing the risk of breast and uterine cancer. However, they have no effect on hot flashes, so are of little help if you are struggling with this symptom. They are more promising if you want to counteract the long-term health risk of osteoporosis without taking a hormone that carries the risk of breast cancer.

The SERM called raloxifene (trade name Evista) is a once-daily tablet. It has been shown to increase bone density and reduce the risk of bone fractures in the spine. The long-term effect of Evista on the risk for breast cancer is unknown at present.

Hormone replacement therapy (HRT)

Your bones can benefit from HRT but only if it is taken long-term. The Framingham Study (a long-term American health research project begun in 1948) revealed in 1993 that:

- Only women who had taken HRT for at least seven years had significantly higher bone mineral density than women who had not taken it.
- The bone mineral density of HRT users declined rapidly as soon as they stopped taking HRT.

- Even seven years of therapy might be insufficient to protect women 75 years and older from fracture.

Calcium supplements

These may be advisable if you cannot obtain your recommended daily intake through food and drink (see the chart on page 47 for the calcium content of common foods).

Vitamin D/calcitonins

Vitamin D supplements are recommended for people with vitamin D deficiency as related to poor diet or limited exposure to sunlight, (e.g., over age 65 and housebound or living in an institution). Remember, however, that excessive exposure to sun can cause skin cancer.

Calcitrol (trade names Rocaltrol and Calcijex) helps to increase the amount of calcium absorption in the digestive tract and increase the amount of calcium that enters the bone.

SIMPLE SOLUTIONS

In 2001, a randomized controlled trial in Melbourne, Australia, explored three interventions to prevent falls among people 70 years and older, half of whom lived alone. The three interventions were group-based exercise, home hazard management, and vision improvement.

Balance measures improved significantly among the exercise group, but all three interventions produced an estimated 14 percent reduction in the annual fall rate.

In this picture you can clearly see the effects of osteoporosis on the spine.

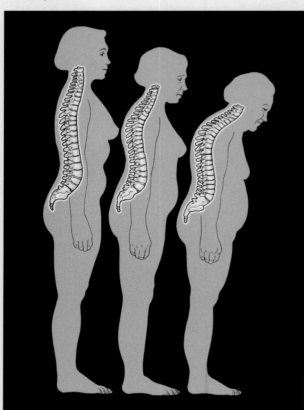

My mother is only 69 years old, yet she has a hunchback (kyphosis) that results in severe back pain and prevents her from sitting for long periods of time. She has lost 2¼" (6 cm) in height, has problems finding suitable clothing, and can wear only sports shoes to prevent possible falls. She was diagnosed as suffering from severe osteoporosis nearly 20 years after the onset of her menopause. I am not taking any chances. I take HRT and daily calcium supplements and undergo bone density testing every two years.

SARAH

PREVENTING FALLS

Most of the fractures associated with osteoporosis are caused by falls. A third of people over the age of 60 have a fall at least once a year, and although not all falls are serious, many result in fractures, especially in older women with osteoporosis.

The chart below describes some of the most common reasons for falls and provides suggestions for ways to prevent such falls.

WHO IS AT RISK?

Most hip fractures occur in people age 80 or older and cause high morbidity and mortality. It is therefore desirable to identify those individuals at greatest risk because that risk can be roughly halved with effective treatment.
Ignac Fogelman, Professor of Nuclear Medicine, Guy's Hospital, London

COMMON REASONS FOR FALLS

Reasons	Prevention
Poor balance caused by weak muscles, low blood pressure, ear problems, or other conditions	• *Exercise keeps muscles strong and improves balance.*
Poor eyesight making it harder to notice hazards, such as a trailing cord or a bump in the sidewalk	• *Make sure you have good lighting in your home.* • *Get an annual eye test.* • *Avoid glare by wearing good-quality sunglasses.*
Footwear	• *Be sure your shoes fit well.*
Hazards at home (where most falls occur)	• *Floor surfaces (mats, carpets, rugs) should lie flat without curled-up edges.* • *Make sure electrical cords are not likely to trip anyone.*
Lighting	• *Have clear lighting with easily accessible switches in all areas of your home.*
Bathroom	• *Have railings fitted to help you in and out of the shower or bathtub and when using the toilet.* • *Use nonslip mats to avoid slippery wet surfaces.*
Hazards outside the home	• *Be aware of uneven pavements, slippery shopping center floors, steep curbs, etc.* • *Keep your yard free of clutter including fallen branches and hoses.*

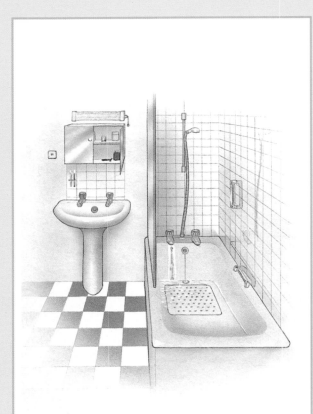

BATHROOM SAFETY

There are some simple precautions you can take to avoid falls in the bathroom. Install hand rails for getting in and out of the bath and always use a nonslip bathmat.

SUMMARY

If you have experienced an early menopause or prolonged amenorrhea (i.e., abnormal suppression or absence of menstruation other than because of pregnancy) or if you have a family history of osteoporosis or are taking corticosteroids, a bone scan is helpful in reaching a decision about treatment.

Explore all your options for maintaining healthy bones for the rest of your life. If you care for your bones, then your bones will take care of you.

At the age of 49, I had a full hysterectomy as a result of cancer. In my late 50s, I broke several ribs falling over a box, and then I broke several other ribs ten years later. In 1995, at the age of 63, I fell off a ladder and broke a leg, fractured my sternum, cracked my collar-bone, chipped an elbow, and again broke four ribs. It was only then I was diagnosed with osteoporosis when a bone density scan showed I was at extreme risk of fracture of my hips and spine.

My doctor put me on a program of daily medication to build up my bone mass, which I've kept up for the last four years. Even so, my bones are still extremely brittle: last week when bringing in the groceries from the car, I used my little finger to lift a plastic supermarket bag containing two cartons of milk and my finger snapped.

For me, living with osteoporosis means:
- *I must be careful all the time.*
- *I must not hurry, especially on uneven surfaces or on rainy days.*
- *I must keep my dog, Gemmi, on a short leash when I walk her each day so that I don't get tangled up and trip.*
- *I must not wear high heels.*
- *I must limit alcohol or better still, abstain, because of its effects on bone density.*
- *I must carry groceries in small amounts, making several trips up 17 stairs.*
- *I must no longer dig the vegetable garden or climb or stretch up to trim trees.*
- *I must only clean things I can reach from floor level.*

Sadly for me, osteoporosis means not being able to run around with my grandchildren. I'm the person sitting on the beach minding the shoes, instead of exploring the rockpools.

BONNIE

HRT and heart disease

If you hold out your hand, palm upward, you see bluish veins under the fine skin of your wrist. These are part of an intricate vascular system circulating blood throughout your body.

A healthy blood supply flows freely, but sometimes blockages occur (as with a blood clot) or plaque forms inside veins, reducing blood flow. If one of these happens to you, you are at risk of suffering either a stroke or a heart attack. These two conditions are part of the group of disorders known as cardiovascular disease (CVD).

Heart and circulatory disease, or CVD, includes all diseases of the heart and blood vessels. The two main diseases in this category are coronary heart disease (CHD) and stroke, but CVD also includes congenital heart disease (i.e., heart deformities present at birth), valvular heart disease, and a range of other diseases of the heart and blood vessels. Both CHD and stroke are caused by blockage in an artery.

Coronary heart disease (CHD) comes in two main forms: angina and heart attack. The latter is also known as a myocardial infarction.

- Angina is caused by a narrowing of the blood vessels to the heart muscle. It is experienced as a pain in the chest brought on by exercise or emotion. It can be mild or severe and generally lasts less than 10 minutes.
- A heart attack causes similar pain but lasts longer and can be fatal. A heart attack results when a blood vessel is entirely blocked by a blood clot.

Cardiovascular disease is a more common cause of morbidity and mortality for women in most countries

High blood pressure Blood pressure is the pressure of the blood in your arteries, which carry blood away from your heart to the rest of your body. High blood pressure happens if the walls of the larger arteries lose their elasticity and become rigid and the smaller vessels contract or become narrowed. People with high blood pressure run a higher risk of having a stroke or heart attack.

Peripheral arterial disease This happens when the arteries that supply blood to the legs become narrowed or completely blocked. Other arteries, such as those supplying blood to the heart and neck, are also likely to be affected.

Diabetes and heart disease These are two of the world's most common chronic diseases. An estimated 5.7 million American women have diabetes.

Blood cholesterol There are two types of cholesterol: dietary and blood. Dietary is contained in food, while blood cholesterol is the amount circulating in the body. Cholesterol is manufactured in the liver and can be deposited in the artery walls by a process called atherosclerosis, which leads to narrowing and hardening of the arteries and then to heart disease.

of the world than osteoporosis and cancer combined. It is unusual for cardiovascular events to occur in women before 60.

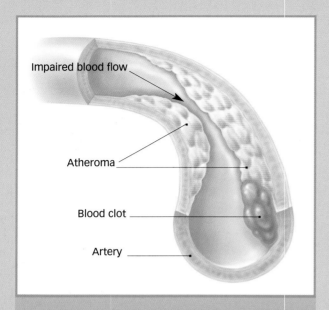

Impaired blood flow

Atheroma

Blood clot

Artery

BLOCKED ARTERIES

The process of coronary heart disease (CHD) begins when the coronary arteries become narrowed by a gradual build-up of fatty material (atheroma) within their walls.

High blood pressure or high cholesterol levels in midlife, and in particular the combination of these risks, increases the risk of Alzheimer's disease in later life by inducing atherosclerosis and thus impairing blood flow to the brain.

DID YOU KNOW?

CVD claims the lives of nearly one million Americans each year. The risk for women rises sharply if their menopause is caused by hysterectomy or oophorectomy.

RISK FACTORS

The following factors place you at high risk of CVD (cardiovascular disease):

- High blood pressure, which is the most important risk factor for a stroke
- A family history of heart disease
- Obesity, which is defined as having a body mass index (BMI) of 30 or higher. A BMI of 26 or higher classifies you as overweight (see the formula for measuring your BMI on page 56).
- A sedentary lifestyle
- Cigarette smoking, which is consistently associated with peripheral arterial disease
- Psychosocial factors, such as stressful situations, depression, and social isolation, have been linked to increased risk.
- Diabetes
- High blood cholesterol, which is associated with cardiovascular disease

The combined effect of two or more risk factors is more powerful than any one risk factor, and some risk factors commonly occur together. For example, screening for diabetes may be appropriate in women with high blood pressure.

THE HEART OF THE MATTER

As we get older, our pattern of risk changes. On average, women acquire heart disease about ten years later than men. Coronary heart disease rates become more similar in men and women as they age, but this reflects a deceleration in male rates of heart disease during middle age, rather than an acceleration in women's postmenopausal rates.

A huge amount of research has been conducted on men and heart disease, but CVD in women is underresearched and underdiagnosed, so that comparatively little is known about it. For years it has been assumed women are

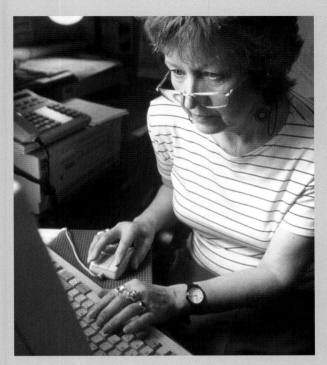

A sedentary lifestyle can place you at risk of heart disease, If your job requires you to sit at a desk all day then make sure that the rest of your life isn't so sedentary.

protected from heart disease as long as estrogen is produced, because this has a beneficial effect on blood cholesterol metabolism. It therefore followed that women lost that protection after the menopause because of the loss of estrogen, resulting in increased risk.

As discussed in Chapter 1, women do indeed lose estrogen during the menopausal years—approximately 40 percent of it—but estrogen continues to be produced in variable quantities for up to 20 years after the menopause.

The observation that the progression of CVD in women is more rapid after the menopause led to the hypothesis that maintaining estrogen levels with HRT could prevent it. Indeed, since the 1970s, more than 30 case-control and prospective studies have reported less heart disease in women using estrogen.

CVD IS LARGELY PREVENTABLE

This has been successfully demonstrated by a community-wide heart health program carried out in the Finnish region of North Karelia, where over a period of 20 years CVD mortality fell by about 70 percent.

TOO MANY BROKEN HEARTS

CVD accounts for more than half of all deaths in Europe of people under age 75, with a total of four million lives taken every year. The Greeks smoke the most and have the biggest problem with CVD; the Portuguese exercise the least and have the highest death rate from stroke in the European Union; the Irish are the most likely to die from coronary heart disease (CHD).

My life changed completely when I was 50 years old. I was sent abroad on business, and on my return, was hospitalized for investigations into persistent vomiting and diarrhea. At the time, I smoked and was also stressed out with my job.

I had a stroke while in the hospital, which the doctor blamed on HRT. I don't think this was true as I had been on it for five years with no problems. Not long afterwards, I suffered my first bout of epilepsy.

In the next couple of years, I became very depressed, confused, and moody and was so relieved when my doctor again prescribed HRT. I am now 61 years old and have been taking HRT for nine years. All of my symptoms have vanished.

LAURA

Body mass index

The amount of body fat you carry may be more significant than your weight alone. The Body Mass Index (BMI) expresses the relationship between a person's weight and height. It is calculated as weight in pounds, divided by height in inches squared. The best way to determine a good weight range for you is to use the BMI formula—you will find a calculator helpful in working it out. Your BMI should fall somewhere between 18 and 25. To be either below 18 or above 25 is to put your health at risk.

Watch your weight during this menopausal transition, as any excess could affect your heart.

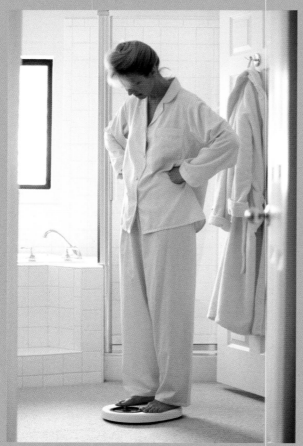

CALCULATING YOUR BODY MASS INDEX

Here is the way to work out your BMI:

Method:

1. Multiply your present weight (in pounds) by 704. This is X.
2. Multiply your height (in inches) by your height (in inches). This is Y.
3. Divide X by Y.

Example:

Let's say you are 5 feet 4 inches (64 inches) tall and weigh 142 pounds.

Multiply 142 by 704—this totals 99,968.

Next, multiply 64 by 64 for a total of 4,096.

Divide 99,968 by 4,096 to result in a BMI of around 24.

You are within a healthy range, although near the high end, and you should be aware that if you gain 10 pounds, your BMI will be in the unhealthy range.

However, one meta-analysis of 22 randomized trials before 1997 that compared HRT with placebo, no therapy, or supplemental vitamins and minerals in predominantly healthy postmenopausal women showed no overall cardioprotective effect of HRT.

The study most often quoted to back up these claims formed part of the Nurses Health Study (see page 43) which found a decreased risk of major or fatal heart disease in estrogen users. But closer examination of the coronary risk factors of this study revealed that this decrease had little to do with the fact that the women were taking HRT. It had far more to do with the reality of their composition as a group: they were a self-selected group of healthy women with less severe vascular risk in

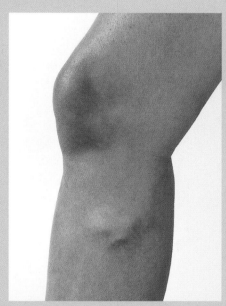

Severe varicose veins are a predisposing factor in the risk of developing a blood clot.

the first place, and they were women who had a commitment to preventive medicine in general.

Estrogen was not keeping these women healthy; rather, healthy women were taking estrogen. And indeed all women in HRT studies are generally better educated, financially comfortable, and enjoying healthier lifestyles.

HRT SEEMS NOT TO PROTECT WOMEN FROM FURTHER HEART ATTACKS

This was the conclusion in 1998 of the first randomized controlled trial large enough to examine the effects of HRT on CVD outcomes. Researchers from 18 medical centers in the USA contributed to a study of 2,763 postmenopausal women with known heart disease whose health was followed for an average of four years. The Heart and Estrogen/Progestogen Replacement Study (HERS) found that the overall rate of cardiovascular events did not differ between the women taking HRT and those taking placebo.

However, an increased risk of venous thromboembolic disease was observed consistently during each year of HERS.

Past perceptions about appropriate indications for the use of HRT were based almost entirely on clinical experience and observational data. These perceptions are being questioned as new knowledge emerges as a result of clinical trials.

> My hot flashes persisted for five to six years after the menopause, even though I was taking HRT. It is difficult to say what benefits it has bought me: my skin has always been clear and my hair glossy, but because I smoke, I think it has protected my heart.
>
> JEAN

DID YOU KNOW?
One clinical trial showed that a "Mediterranean diet" supplemented with alpha-linoleic acid found in seeds and nuts significantly reduced the risk of recurrent coronary events in patients with heart disease.

VITAMIN E

A study by scientists at Cambridge University and Papworth Hospital, UK, in 1996 found that a daily dose of vitamin E reduced the risk of having a heart attack by 75 percent. This 18-month double-blind controlled trial involved 2,000 patients with coronary atherosclerosis (see box, page 53). The number of heart attacks in the group taking the vitamin E was a quarter of that in the group taking placebo.

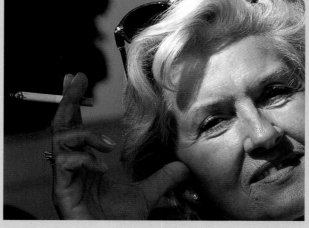

If you smoke you are more at risk of heart disease.

CURRENT PERCEPTIONS

Although current thinking on this issue is that HRT protects against coronary disease, the randomized clinical trials reported so far have shown no benefit for reducing further coronary events. Similarly, although it is said that, unlike oral contraceptives, HRT does not increase the risk of venous thromboembolism (a blood clot), clinical trials have confirmed a threefold increased risk of venous thromboembolism in women taking HRT.

The risk of blood clot appears to be greatest during the first year of HRT use, and predisposing factors are:

- A personal or family history of venous thromboembolism.
- Recent surgery or trauma.
- Obesity.
- Severe varicose veins.
- Prolonged immobilization.

Heart disease is a degenerative disease linked to lifestyle factors. When it occurs it is because problems have been building up for years.

REDUCING YOUR RISK

There are many dietary and lifestyle changes that you can make to reduce your risk of cardiovascular disease.

- Include more oily fish, nuts, seeds, and oils in your meals. The essential fatty acids in these foods are important for the prevention of heart disease. Eating fish three times a week reduces the risk of CVD because fish oils lower cholesterol, thin your blood, and reduce the risk of narrowing of the arteries.
- Try to stay within an appropriate weight range for your height and frame.
- Stop smoking cigarettes and avoid "passive" smoking situations.

ISCHEMIC HEART DISEASE

"Ischemia" is an inadequate supply of blood and is a consequence of the gradual narrowing of the coronary arteries that supply the blood and oxygen to the muscles of the heart.

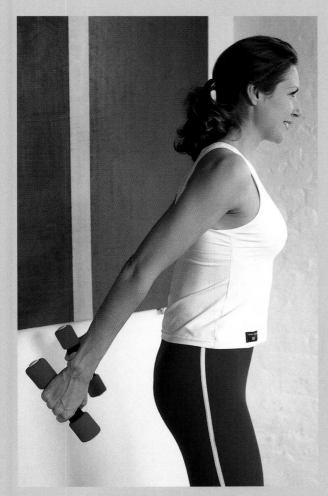
You can maintain muscle mass with these handheld weights by training for at least 1 hour a week.

- Eat more soy products. Soy beans are a complete protein and contain all eight essential amino acids.
- Eat more fresh vegetables and fruit, as well as dried fruit. Fiber in potatoes, carrots, apples, beans, and oats binds up the cholesterol and carries it out of your body.
- Take vitamin E supplements.
- If you have a disability that prevents you from taking active exercise, try to arrange regular physiotherapy, massage, and hydrotherapy sessions.

RAW FOOD FOR A HEALTHY HEART
An ambitious study conducted between 1973 and 1979 recruited 11,000 British men and women from among the customers of health food shops and other people with an interest in health foods and vegetarianism.

Its aim was to examine the relationship between six dietary factors (a vegetarian diet and consumption of wholegrain bread, bran cereals, nuts and dried fruit, fresh fruit, and raw salad) and mortality for which associations with diet have been suggested.

The most significant association found after a 17-year follow-up was that daily consumption of raw salad was associated with a 26 percent reduction in death from ischemic heart disease (see box, opposite), slightly greater than that for fresh fruit (24 percent).

SUMMARY
Help yourself to a decision about this issue by:

- Assessing your risk of CVD.
- Reducing risk by eliminating two or more of your risk factors.
- Improving your lifestyle and adopting healthier eating habits .
- Protecting your heart with regular weight-bearing exercise.
- Recognizing that HRT cannot prevent CVD.

Remember, if you have already suffered a heart attack or stroke, HRT will not protect you against another occurrence.

The special case of diabetes

Diabetes is one of the world's two most common chronic diseases, and more than 10 million people in the US have the disease. Diabetic women are at greatly increased risk of developing ischemic heart disease.

Diabetes mellitis is a condition in which the amount of glucose (sugar) in the blood is too high because the body cannot use it properly.

Glucose comes from the digestion of starchy foods such as bread, rice, and potatoes, as well as from sugar and other sweet foods. It is also produced in the liver.

There are two main types of diabetes :

- Type 1 diabetes, also known as insulin-dependent diabetes, usually appears before the age of 40.
- Type 2 diabetes, also known as noninsulin-dependent diabetes, is more common among women after, rather than before, the menopause.

Type 1 diabetes develops if the body is unable to produce any insulin (a hormone produced by the pancreas), and it

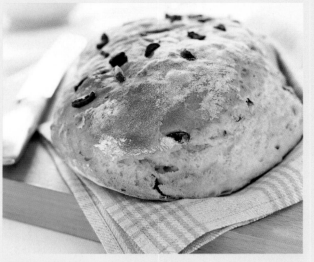

Bread is a universal staple food containing complex carbohydrates.These are an important source of energy.

is treated by insulin injections. Dietary changes are essential. Type 2 diabetes (late onset in midlife or older) develops when the body can still produce some insulin, but not enough, or when the insulin that is produced does not work properly. It is treated either by diet and exercise alone; by diet, exercise, and tablets; or by diet, exercise, and insulin injections.

The risk of death from CVD is five times greater in women age 50 to 60 who have diabetes than in women of the same age who do not. Coronary heart disease (CHD) is a major cause of morbidity and mortality in postmenopausal women who have type 2 (non-insulin-dependent) diabetes. Furthermore, the Framingham Study (as mentioned on pages 49 to 50) showed a sixfold increase in sudden cardiac death in female compared with male diabetic patients.

In 1998, a British study showed that type 2 diabetic postmenopausal women were 30 percent less likely to be prescribed HRT, compared with nondiabetic women. The reason for this reluctance to prescribe is unclear, but it seems to be driven by a perception that

DIABETES AND OSTEOPOROSIS

Women with with type 1 diabetes have reduced bone density, which can be demonstrated after a few years of insulin treatment. While it is known that insulin is important for the growth of bone cells and mineral metabolism, the exact mechanism of the osteopenia of diabetes is not fully understood.

Women who have type 2 diabetes have increased bone turnover but normal bone density.

HRT will increase thromboembolic events and cause a deterioration in glucose tolerance.

In the future, it may well be that all women with diabetes should take HRT to reduce their risk of CVD. However, the appropriate studies have not yet been done. Indeed, there are no long-term studies of women with diabetes, and no studies at all on women with type 1 diabetes.

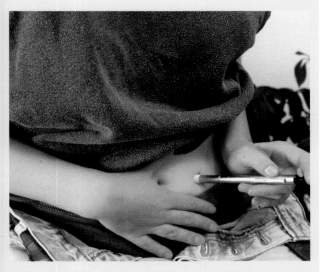

Type 1 diabetes is treated by insulin injections, but you may not need injections if you suffer from Type 2 diabetes.

A surgical menopause

If you have had a hysterectomy (removal of the womb) and/or oophorectomy (removal of the ovaries), you are likely to be prescribed HRT after surgery. This will be for various reasons, depending on your age and on why you needed the surgery. HRT would be recommended for you:

- If you are a young woman (20 to 30 years of age) having a hysterectomy and oophorectomy, and are likely to experience severe menopausal symptoms after the operation.
- If you are young (20 to 30 years of age) and having an oophorectomy, which will cause an artificial menopause and an increased risk of osteoporosis.
- If you are near menopause (45 to 50 years of age) undergoing hysterectomy because you may experience menopausal symptoms.
- If you are near to menopause (48 to 52 years of age) and undergoing hysterectomy and oophorectomy.

In addition, if you are nearing menopause, postmenopausal, and/or disabled, HRT often is recommended to alleviate menopausal symptoms and avoid possible osteoporosis.

DIABETES AND HRT
There is no evidence that short-term treatment using HRT to relieve menopausal symptoms is unsafe for women with diabetes. In most women, there is no effect on insulin requirements, but occasionally a little more insulin may be needed to maintain good control of glucose levels. The use of HRT on a long-term basis is much more controversial.

ONE IN FOUR
In 25 percent of women who have had their wombs removed, the ovaries become less efficient, and premature menopause sets in within two years. The exact cause of this is unknown, but it could be due to a loss of blood supply to the ovaries or the development of thick adhesions around the ovaries following hysterectomy.

The missing hormone: natural progesterone

In the early 1900s, research into the mysteries of women's hormones first revealed the existence of estrogen. Further investigations identified a second hormone that was necessary to maintain a successful pregnancy: this was named progesterone (i.e., pro-gestation).

Since then, research into menopausal problems has concentrated almost exclusively on the perceived loss of estrogen, and little attention has been paid to the decline in progesterone, since it was believed that its main purpose was to help reproductive function.

There is now a body of opinion that has challenged this assumption. It is spearheaded by a doctor who has contributed hugely to our knowledge of hormones by bringing the issue of the use of progesterone before the medical world.

IN THE BEGINNING...

In 1994, an American doctor addressed 125 fellow medical practitioners at a meeting in a London hospital. His topic was the hormone progesterone.

A family practitioner for 30 years, John Lee had become increasingly concerned about his aging osteoporotic patients who were unable to take estrogen because they already had breast cancer, diabetes, or vascular disorders. He realized he could encourage them to adopt a more healthy lifestyle, but that was not enough to counter the osteoporosis.

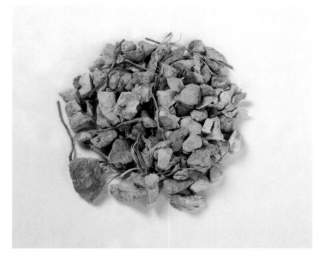

Mexican wild yam (*Dioscorea villosa*) contains a substance called diosgenin.

His meeting with Dr. Ray Peat, a biochemist from Oregon, at a medical seminar in 1978 had changed his life. Years of research had convinced Dr. Peat that progesterone was a very important hormone for osteoporotic postmenopausal women, for while estrogen slowed bone loss, the function of progesterone was to increase the formation of new bone. Furthermore, he claimed progesterone could be made from yams, soy, and indeed 5,000 different plants.

Astonished and excited by these claims, Dr. Lee pursued them further, researching back to 1938 when Dr. Russell Marker found plants contained fats and oils called saponins, which he then discovered could be converted into "natural" progesterone. In general, saponins are thought to be cholesterol-lowering agents.

During the following three years, Dr. Lee monitored 100 postmenopausal white women ranging in age from 38 to 83 years (an average age of 65), using a program of low-protein vegetable diet, modest exercise, and vitamin supplementation, plus a transdermal dose of progesterone.

Regular bone density tests (at six-month or yearly

> Four years ago menopausal symptoms such as mood swings, forgetfulness, lack of focus, vaginal dryness, and discomfort were driving me crazy. My family medical history contraindicated HRT. Mum had high blood pressure and a stroke when she was 60, and I had had a breast lump and a malignant melanoma on my wrist. I read about progesterone in a health magazine and, within days, was using a progesterone cream. I think it is fantastic; it has regulated all the problems I had.
>
> FIONA

TESTING TIMES

After three months of treatment for menopausal symptoms in a double-blind placebo-controlled study using a topical product containing wild yam, researchers at the Baker Medical Research Institute, Melbourne, Australia, found no statistical difference between placebo and active creams, even though "mood swings" of women using the active cream actually improved in this trial. The ingredient responsible for this may well have been the geranium essential oil used in the cream.

intervals) revealed:

- A reversal of osteoporosis with some women actually gaining bone density.
- An increase of bone density in the lumbar region.

Not only had their bones improved, but the progesterone treatment had other benefits: the women felt better, they had less breast swelling and tenderness, their low thyroid problems improved, their high blood pressure went down, and they showed a return to normal libido.

The results appeared to have potential, and before long the commercial bandwagon swung into action. Huge farms growing wild yams sprang up in Mexico, and various steroidal saponins and other plant compounds were studied. It was found that one of the richest sources for commercial use was a substance called diosgenin in the Mexican wild yam (*Dioscorea villosa*)—not to be confused with the average supermarket yam, which is really a sweet potato. *Dioscorea* species have been used as remedies for at least 5,000 years for conditions ranging from rheumatoid arthritis and colic to dysmenorrhea (difficult or painful menstruation).

It was the easy and inexpensive conversion of diosgenin

into a molecule that is identical to the progesterone hormone made by the body that paved the way for natural progesterone creams (or gels) that could be smeared on any soft skin, such as a woman's tummy, inner thigh, or breast.

While relief from menopausal symptoms found some support, the idea that progesterone could increase bone density was received with some skepticism.

In one way, this is heartening, given that estrogen was once marketed as a "wonder drug" without any knowledge of its side-effects or long-term consequences. But in another way it is anything but heartening. There have been few clinical trials to support these claims, and indeed Dr. Lee's conclusion to his article titled *Osteoporosis reversal—the role of progesterone* in which he states that "It does not require a double-blind placebo controlled experiment to conclude that progesterone is of great benefit in treating and preventing osteoporosis" hardly helped further his cause.

Whatever his humanitarian desire to help those women who could not take HRT, there remained a fundamental question about the results of his surveys, since there was no control group not taking progesterone for comparison.

HOW MUCH SHOULD I USE?

Most doctors suggest a quarter to half a teaspoon a day. You need to monitor how rapidly it is absorbed. If your symptoms increase, use more; if your symptoms decrease, use less.

HOW LONG DO I HAVE TO USE IT TO SEE RESULTS?

This varies enormously. Some women notice relief from hot flashes almost immediately. In general, menopausal difficulties will be relieved within three months.

WILL IT HELP VAGINAL DRYNESS?

Natural progesterone cream used on the perineum (that is the area between your vulva and anus) and intra-vaginally is generally successful in treating both vaginal dryness and vulvar dystrophy (shrinkage of the vaginal tissues). You might prefer to apply oil intravaginally—for example, by putting a few drops of it on your finger and inserting this into the vagina.

CAN I USE THE CREAM CONTINUOUSLY AFTER THE MENOPAUSE?

When you are postmenopausal, use progesterone cream for two or three weeks a month, then discontinue for a week so that at least 5 to 7 days a month remain hormone-free.

ARE THERE ANY SIDE-EFFECTS TO USING NATURAL PROGESTERONE?

No, it is not known to have any side-effects except for altering the menstrual cycle temporarily in some women and bringing about feelings of euphoria.

Very occasionally, a postmenopausal woman will have a short period for the first month or two, then this stops permanently. Should this happen, it is a sign that the

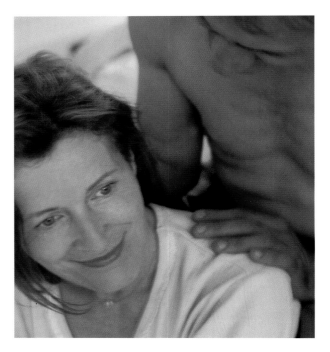

Testosterone contributes to sex drive and feelings of energy and well-being.

progesterone is causing your body to eliminate excess stored estrogen that triggers shedding of the endometrium or breakthrough bleeding. If any kind of breakthrough bleeding continues for more than three months, it is important to consult a doctor.

Some doctors resist prescribing natural progesterone as a part of HRT because they feel uncomfortable about the lack of studies done on its ability to make the necessary changes in the uterus. Yet you may be someone who cannot tolerate synthetic progestogen, especially if you have a genetic tendency towards PMS. If that is so, you may need to take higher, more frequent doses of natural progesterone than if you used a synthetic progestogen.

Testosterone for women

In his research over the years, Dr. Lee discovered that progesterone is used throughout our bodies—nerves, brain cells, thyroid gland, fat metabolism, and muscle building. He also investigated the effects of testosterone.

Although testosterone is known as the "male" hormone because men have much higher levels, women also produce it. Testosterone contributes to bone and muscle strength, sex drive, and feelings of energy and well-being.

In women, most testosterone is produced by the stroma, a part of the ovary, and levels are fairly consistent throughout the menstrual cycle, with perhaps a slight midcycle surge that increases your sex drive when you ovulate. Levels often begin to decline when women are in their late 30s or early 40s and can decrease as much as 50 percent following the menopause. Symptoms of low testosterone levels include:

- A low sex drive, muscle weakness, and loss of a feeling of well-being.
- Low energy, irritability, forgetfulness, crying spells, and hot flashes that do not respond to estrogen alone.
- Headaches or migraines.

The role of testosterone in depression is a focus of current research, and positive effects of testosterone therapy on mood in naturally menopausal women have been reported.

WHAT TREATMENT IS AVAILABLE?

Testosterone can be administered in the form of injection, pills, or cream. Soy-based natural testosterone is available in tablets, pellets, and injections, as well as gels and creams. The latter have greater absorption, produce more stable blood levels, and bypass the liver.

WILL I GROW A BEARD?

Low-dose testosterone treatment needs to be carefully monitored. It can improve sexual response, but doctors

---

DID YOU KNOW?
Studies in the United States showed an increase in frequency of sexual activity, orgasmic pleasure, and positive well-being when transdermal testosterone was used for 12 weeks by 75 women aged from 31 to 56 with impaired sexual functioning after surgically induced menopause (hysterectomy and oophorectomy).

are often reluctant to prescribe it because of its side-effects. These include acne and virilization (enlargement of the clitoris and deepening of the voice), as well as that most feared of all—hirsutism (excessive hair growth), which occurs in 5 to 20 percent of women. Fortunately this effect is reversible and usually disappears when the dose is reduced.

Summary

Hormone replacement therapy using estrogen and progestogen offers short-term risks and benefits for the alleviation of menopausal symptoms. It also offers long-term benefits if you are at risk of certain conditions plus associated risks.

Progesterone cream appears to alleviate menopausal symptoms, but as yet there is only anecdotal evidence to indicate its beneficial effects on bones and no evidence on possible heart benefits.

A low dose of testosterone has been shown to improve libido and is especially important if the ovaries have been surgically removed.

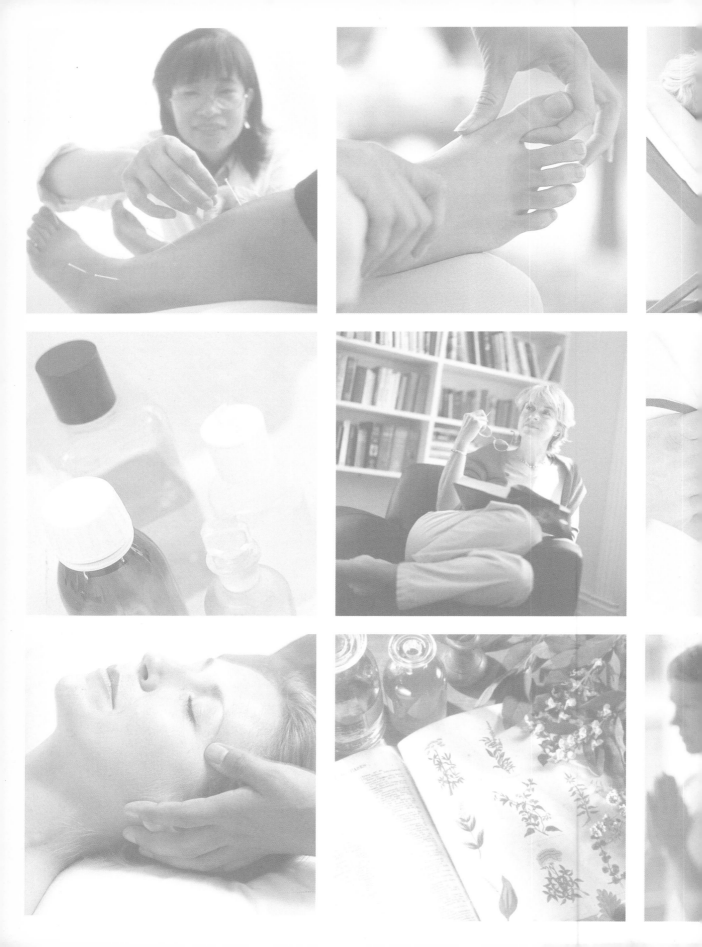

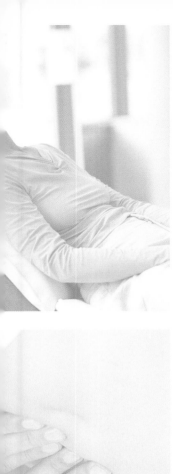

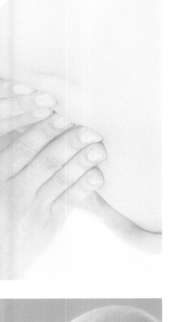

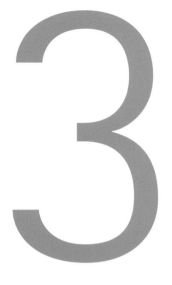

3

Alternatives
to HRT

Considering the alternatives

Having read the preceding chapters, you should have a better idea about hormone replacement therapy and your own unique risks and benefits. Now you can weigh whether or not it is right for you.

Your decision may be an easy one. For example, your menopausal symptoms are bothersome, especially your memory, which is all over the place. You have always known you were at risk of osteoporosis because your mother and grandmother both suffered from it, and you now realize that HRT is also likely to protect you from Alzheimer's disease, which your father had. You do not particularly welcome the idea of continuing monthly "bleeds" until you have had no periods for a year but feel this is a small price to pay for the benefits of HRT.

Maybe your decision is not so clear-cut. You can cope with hot flashes in the daytime, but your night sweats are horrendous, and their impact is badly affecting both your domestic and working life. You now realize you are not at risk of osteoporosis but decide to have regular bone scans, just to be on the safe side. Your family medical history shows no evidence of strokes, heart attacks, bowel cancer, or Alzheimer's disease. In view of these factors, you decide to give HRT a try but only as a temporary measure.

Perhaps you are a woman with a disability that requires using a wheelchair. You have been feeling low and depressed and wonder if it is hormonally based. You have had a few hot flashes over the last few weeks, your concentration is not as sharp as usual, and you seem overtaken by chronic tiredness. You are reluctant to consider HRT because there is breast cancer in your family, so you decide to wait and see if any other menopausal symptoms appear. Because you lead a mainly sedentary life, you are a little concerned about being at risk of either a heart attack or stroke, and decide to increase your physiotherapy sessions and explore the possibility of hydrotherapy.

Or perhaps you believe any chemical interference in this transitional stage of your life is "medicalizing" a normal happening. Nothing you have read in this book so far has changed your mind. Equally, you are not happy to simply "grin and bear" your menopausal symptoms; you realize something must be done, as your moods and irritability at work have led to a tearful confrontation with colleagues. You resolve to explore alternative ways of helping yourself through this unsettling time.

Natural alternatives

Every day, thousands of us seek help from acupuncturists, chiropractors, osteopaths, herbalists, and homeopaths as well as practitioners of other therapies, such as

Alternatives to HRT may alleviate menopausal symptoms and help you to feel fitter and more relaxed.

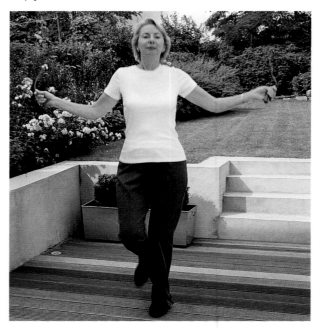

reflexology and aromatherapy. Why should there be such interest in complementary medicine given the extraordinary achievements of orthodox medicine? It would be hard to exaggerate the benefits that have been obtained by applying scientific principles to medicine: most bacterial infections are curable, smallpox has been wiped out worldwide, and polio has ceased to be a major problem, at least in Western countries. Almost every week the media relays enthusiastic accounts of medical techniques or discoveries, such as organ transplantation; in vitro fertilization and "test-tube" babies; hip, knee, and even arm replacements; cures for many cancers; and gene therapy.

And yet the fact is that much of this is divorced from the daily lives of most people. For women, it is often menstrual disorders that badly affect their lives, often presenting as depression, headaches, backache, water retention, and premenstrual syndrome (PMS). The end result of an average six-minute interview with a harassed general practitioner is most likely to be a prescription for antidepressants, painkillers, tranquilizers, or sleeping tablets. Some of these are helpful in the short term, but many do not provide solutions and some even carry the potential risks of addiction and side-effects. In view of this, it is highly unlikely a therapy such as HRT could offer a universal panacea to women struggling through the "change" from their reproductive to their postreproductive years.

The fact that doctors are unable to guarantee the safety of prescribed drugs was all too clearly exemplified by the thalidomide tragedy in the late 1950s, when thousands of women who were given a drug to counteract morning sickness in pregnancy gave birth to children with severe limb deformities. Similarly, prescriptions of drugs such as Valium caused its users long-term problems. Medicine has also felt the winds of change blowing through its corridors of power as a climate of accountability has entered the arena. And many patients are much more medically literate than before, both as a direct result of

medical trauma and because of the easy accessibility of information through the Internet.

The combination of suspicion of drugs and disenchantment with orthodox medicine has produced fertile ground for complementary medicine.

For years, the conventional medical community has been less than welcoming of complementary medicine—and with some justification. After all, in many places anyone could rent a room, buy a leather couch, screw up a shiny brass plate outside their door, preferably with a string of impressive-sounding letters after their name—and bingo! they were in business. They could be a real menace and danger to the potential patient. But how was the patient to know that?

The recognition of this problem eventually led many practitioners to put their houses in order: regulations, codes of ethics and competence, and validation now form benchmarks for public confidence and have paved the way for increasing collaboration with the conventional medical professions.

It would be easy to conclude that there is a powerful placebo effect at work, and this attitude is encouraged by the shortage of reliable, responsible research in the field of alternative medicine in some countries, especially given that complementary medicine researchers have to compete with applicants from conventional medicine for funding.

Nevertheless, times are changing. In the United States, a National Center for Complementary and Alternative Medicine (NCCAM) was set up in 1998 to explore these practices in the context of rigorous science, to train complementary and alternative researchers, and disseminate the resultant information to the public and professionals. In March, 2002 a White House Commission released a report promoting the wider use of alternative therapies. The report, which took nearly two years to complete, also called for more research into alternative therapies. The US budget for 2003 includes an estimate for over $100 million for this purpose. Unfortunately, however, they have yet to come up with research evidence into treatment of menopausal symptoms by complementary medicine. This is perhaps surprising in view of the fact that a 1997 study conducted by the North American Menopause Society reported that 30 percent of women use acupuncture, natural estrogen(s), herbal supplements, and phytoestrogens to relieve their menopausal symptoms.

Personal recommendation is one way of choosing a complementary practitioner, so talk to people you know who have tried alternative therapies, and ask how they felt about the treatment they received. What did they think of the practitioner? Was the therapy being practiced in clean and properly equipped premises? How much did the treatment cost, and how often did they receive it? Nowadays, reputable practitioners include information about their membership of professional organizations in their advertisements, and you should always check this out before you make an appointment.

Many complementary practitioners offer time, a sympathetic manner, and therapies that are concerned with the "whole woman." However, this is not always the case and if, after an initial visit, you feel uncomfortable with your practitioner, trust your judgement and do not continue.

In this chapter we explore complementary therapies in relation to the menopause, and you will see how many contain overlapping elements. Some, such as meditation, relaxation, and yoga, are self-help techniques, while acupuncture requires a consultation with a practitioner.

Acupuncture

The use of acupuncture first caught the Western imagination around 1958 when it became recognized for its effectiveness in pain control, primarily for postoperative care. Later, it was introduced as an alternative to anesthesia during operations, first with minor procedures, such as tooth extraction, and later with major operations on the limbs and abdomen.

Unfortunately, this dramatic use of acupuncture led to a widespread misconception. Traditionally, acupuncture has emphasized prevention; to the Chinese, a sick man

Fine, sterile needles are inserted in the skin at relevant points. They can be left in just briefly, or be inserted for about half-an-hour, depending on the condition.

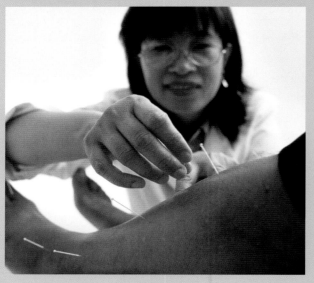

PAIN RELIEF
Legend has it that acupuncture was first discovered by a soldier shot by an arrow. When struck by a second arrow, the soldier reported that the pain from the first wound disappeared.

visiting an acupuncturist is comparable to a thirsty man starting to dig a well.

Acupuncture was first used widely in China, and its history is closely connected with the development of Chinese medicine in general. The theory of Chinese medicine evolved out of an era of philosophical speculation and intense consideration of the nature of life by great thinkers, such as Confucius. Its four methods of diagnosis—observing, listening and smelling, asking, and touching—remain as much the cornerstones of modern-day acupuncture treatment as they were in 200 BC, when a Chinese doctor, Bia Que, brought a prince out of a coma using acupuncture.

Central to the concept of acupuncture is the idea that the body is self-healing; that it is a self-rectifying whole, a network of interrelating and interacting energies. The even distribution and flow of these energies maintains health; any interruption, depletion, or stagnation of energies leads to disease. When this happens, acupuncture tries to aid the natural processes of healing, helping the body to correct itself by a realignment or redirection of energy which the Chinese call Qi (pronounced "chee").

So what is Qi? It is often translated as breath, life-force, or vitality—or simply as that which makes us alive. If there is no Qi, there is no life. Strong and energetic people have plenty of Qi; tired and depressed people lack Qi.

Along with the notion of Qi, acupuncture recognizes a subtle energy system by which Qi is circulated through the body in a network of channels or "meridians." The acupuncture points lie along these meridians and when the acupuncture needle is inserted, it is the Qi that is affected. In some ways the circulation of Qi is similar to the blood circulation and nervous system, although it is invisible to the eye.

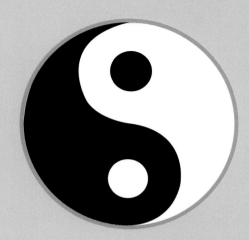

The tai chi symbol shows how yin and yang are opposites, but inseparable.

Accepting this understanding of the body as an energetic and vibrating whole leads to a new approach to health and disease, for it draws together all the diverse signs and symptoms of ill health to form a "pattern of disharmony" that includes the mental and emotional state as much as physical problems.

YIN AND YANG

The idea of harmony and balance form the basis of the concept of "yin" and "yang." The belief that each individual is governed by the opposing but complementary forces of yin and yang is central to all Chinese thought because it is believed to affect everything in the universe.

Traditionally, yin is dark, passive, cold, and negative, while yang is light, active, warm, and positive. We might say they represent opposites, such as happy versus sad, tired versus energetic, cold versus hot.

The tai chi symbol on the previous page illustrates how yin and yang flow into each other, with a little yin always within yang, and a little yang always within yin. The body, mind, and emotions are all subject to these influences: When the two opposing forces are in balance we feel good, but if one force dominates the other, the imbalance can result in ill health.

One of the main aims of the acupuncturist is to restore and maintain the balance of yin and yang.

As you can see, acupuncture is not a system of medicine in isolation. It should be seen as one major method of treatment within a complete system that has a different perspective on health from that of orthodox Western medicine. The idea of treating a patient's headaches in one medical department, their menstrual pains in another, and their insomnia in a third would seem extraordinary to a traditional acupuncturist who believes there must be a common root.

Nowadays, a Westernized branch of acupuncture rejects the existence of channels or "meridians" and believes that acupuncture works by way of the nervous system and that its effects can, in principle, be explained in terms of anatomy and physiology.

You need to decide whether you are going to consult a lay practitioner (someone who may have had no formal training and possesses no accepted academic qualifications) or a doctor who is fully qualified through conventional medical training and who has undergone further training in acupuncture. Both types of practitioner are widely available.

PINPOINTING THE PROBLEM

During your first acupuncture consultation, the practitioner generally asks for details about your general condition. These questions can relate to all your physical, emotional, and energetic signs and symptoms. Although some of

them may seem unrelated, all can help the acupuncturist form a more complete picture of your condition.

The practitioner will also ask to see your tongue. This tongue examination is a very important source of information for the acupuncturist: the shape, color, coating, and texture of the various parts of your tongue yield information about the state of your organs. A healthy tongue should be reddish in color with little or no fur. It should not appear swollen or contracted, neither

Your tongue can reveal a lot about the health of your organs.

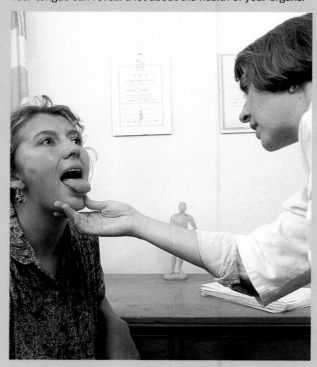

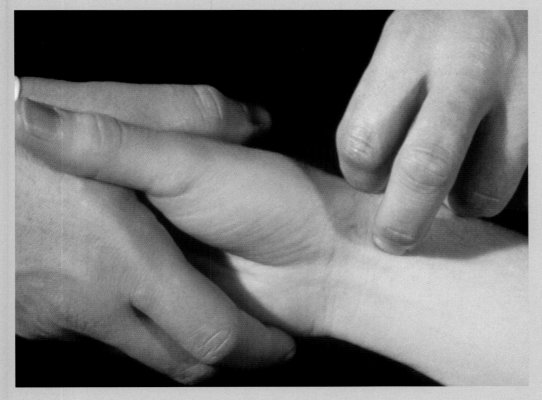

Taking accurate pulse readings on each wrist is a very important part of examination by an acupuncturist.

should there be cracks on the surface or "teeth marks" along its sides.

During the consultation, a full medical history is taken. Other important questions concern:

- Eating and sleep patterns.

- Sensations of heat and cold, perspiration, and whether this occurs during the day or night.
- Headaches—when they occur and in what part of the head.
- Urination and defecation, including frequency of passing urine and any tendency to either constipation or diarrhea.

ACUPUNCTURE AND HOT FLASHES

Between 1995 and 1999 in Staffordshire, United Kingdom, 22 breast cancer patients, aged between 38 and 59, were referred by an oncologist for acupuncture treatment of hot flashes. Analysis of this four-year study revealed that 82 percent experienced effective relief from hot flashes, and all of them recorded some reduction after completion of the course.

SAFETY FIRST

Before undergoing any treatment, you should ask about the sterilization procedures in use at the clinic. In many countries, all registered acupuncturists are required by law to sterilize needles. Disposable needles are available if you prefer, although they will obviously be more expensive.

> *When I was 46, my periods suddenly became much heavier for six months with midcycle bleeding. The doctor diagnosed a fibroid, and a hysterectomy was recommended. I was horrified and asked to see the acupuncturist. I am very fortunate because complementary therapists work on the same premises as my physician, so all I had to do was walk down the corridor and make an appointment. The midcycle bleeding stopped after two treatments, and my periods were normal for about 18 months. Then the midcycle bleeding started again and further treatment alleviated 90 percent of this. By now I had realized I was menopausal, so I continued with acupuncture for another year. During this time, my periods stopped altogether.*
>
> **CAROLINE**

DID YOU KNOW?
The symptoms of just over 50 percent of 300 menopausal women disappeared when treated with acupuncture at the First Hospital, Tianjin, China, in 1998.

If you consult an acupuncturist for treatment of menopausal problems, you will be asked about your menstrual cycles and the menopausal symptoms you have had. You will then be asked to undress, except for your underclothes, so the acupuncturist can examine areas of your body that are painful and to feel for heat, cold, swelling, tightness, or lack of skin tone. Specific acupuncture points may be touched to see if they are painful, particularly points on your abdomen and on each side of your spine.

You may be surprised that the acupuncturist takes your pulse at both wrists and at three positions on the hand, namely, by the index, middle, and ring finger. Acupuncturists believe that they can assess the balance of energy from these three positions and gain the key to your internal state. Your pulses will be checked again at intervals during treatment to monitor the energy changes.

Having gathered together all this information, the acupuncturist formulates the appropriate treatment for you. The choice of acupuncture points differs with each patient. Some points may be used repeatedly until a particular imbalance is corrected.

TREATMENT
Acupuncture stimulates the fine network of nerves running in the skin and sometimes nerves in the deeper tissues as well. These then in turn affect the central nervous system, blocking pain and altering the nervous system's control of other bodily organs. Some patients show very little sensitivity to the needles and do not feel anything when they are inserted. Others may be aware of increased sensitivity in particular areas or on particular meridians. In general, however, treatment should not be painful, and when needle sensation occurs it should not last more than a few seconds. It is usually described as a "tingling" sensation or a feeling of numbness radiating from the needle.

Treatment might be once a week to begin with, then at longer intervals as the condition responds. The treatment schedule depends on you and your "pattern of disharmony." It is demonstrably untrue to say that the results of acupuncture are "all in the mind." After all, treatments have been successfully carried out on very small children and animals. It is unlikely that a cow could be hypnotized into improved health by a veterinary surgeon!

Traditional Chinese medicine

Traditional Chinese medicine incorporates not only acupuncture, but also herbal medicines, dietary suggestions, massage and/or exercises, or lifestyle changes. It would appear that Chinese medicinal herbs are more effective when used in conjunction with the other elements of traditional Chinese medicine.

Because of its holistic view of the body and mind, it is very specific for each patient's needs. For example, five different women coming into a clinic complaining of hot flashes will have a variety of different accompanying signs and symptoms, no two of which are exactly alike. Therefore, each woman will receive an individually tailored treatment plan with different herbs, different acupuncture therapy, and different lifestyle recommendations.

According to traditional Chinese medicine the clinical picture of hot flashes shows a deterioration in the yin of the liver, weakness in the blood of the heart, and an exhaustion of the water of the kidney.

The deficiency of water is countered by an excess of fire, which endangers the control of the yin of the liver and unleashes its yang. There are two pathological mechanisms:

- The combined effects of deficiency in the kidney, hyperactivity in the liver, and flare-up of heart fire will lead to palpitation, insomnia, and dizziness.
- The imbalance between the spleen and liver is manifested by emotional depression, irritability, loss of temper, and an oppressive feeling in the chest.

Medicinal herbs are just one part of Chinese medicine.

CONTRADICTORY EVIDENCE

Chinese herbal medicine has been used for centuries for treating menopausal symptoms, and some clinical trials in China have shown them to be very effective.

But the outcome of a placebo-controlled trial using Chinese medicinal herbs to treat 55 menopausal women in Australia (1998–1999) found the herbs were no more effective than placebo in reducing hot flashes and night sweats.

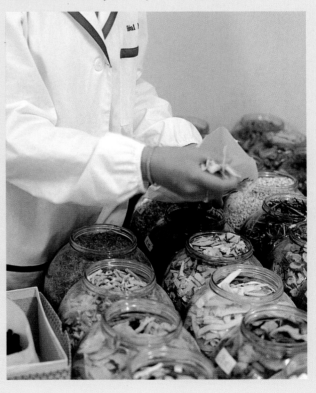

Medical Herbalism

There can be little doubt that plants were the first source of medicines, and the use of herbs as a source of healing remedies is inherent in all cultures in all historical times. Experience taught primitive man that particular leaves could heal a wound caused by an arrowhead, and that some leaves could be boiled to cure a fever. Evidence that the poppy was used to relieve sickness and pain has been found in some early cave dwellings, where poppy seeds were probably used as a sedative.

Over the centuries, plants have been sampled for food and tried as medicine. Who, for example, discovered that a tincture of opium from the poppy would stop children from crying? How did we learn that oil from the beans of the castor tree, in small amounts, made a reliable purgative, but two or three beans themselves would cause death within a few hours? Or that the extracted oil would bring relief when applied to burns and septic wounds and would also make a useful fuel for lamps? Yet both these plants must have been regularly used for these purposes for thousands of years; some of their seeds were found in the ancient tombs of Egypt, dated 1500 BC.

In primitive cultures, this information was so important to the community that it was put in the care of a caste of priests/physicians. Medicine became closely associated with magic, religion, and astrology. Then in 460 BC, the Hippocratic school attempted to separate herbal medicine from the occult and relate it to careful observation of the patient. It was Hippocrates who formulated the principle that treatment and dosage should be decided in accordance with the individual patient's requirement. This is one of the cornerstones of modern-day medical herbalism, as is the belief that the whole plant should be prescribed. Herbalists believe the whole plant is balanced by nature in such a fashion as to make it a much safer remedy than extracted parts.

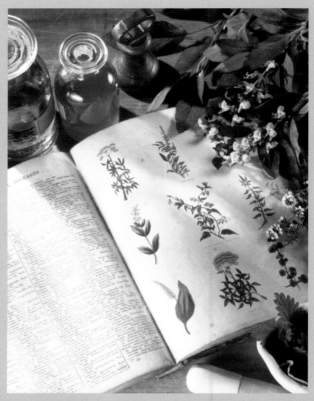

Many different herbs are used to make up the complex herbal preparations that are the mainstay of medical herbalism.

The herbal remedies of antiquity became more accessible to more people with the advent of printing during the Renaissance, but then the dawn of scientific medicine in the seventeenth century, with its emphasis on reason and experiment, challenged these doctrines. The herbalists' ancient authority was further undermined by the emergence of inorganic remedies, and herbal remedies were increasingly sidelined.

However, in every rural community since prehistory there were likely to be individuals, mostly women ("wise women") who were regarded as specialists in the art of using healing plants. They satisfied the needs of basic health care, treating injuries and illness and usually acting as midwives as well. Many of these women were tied to a larger network of women's culture that handed

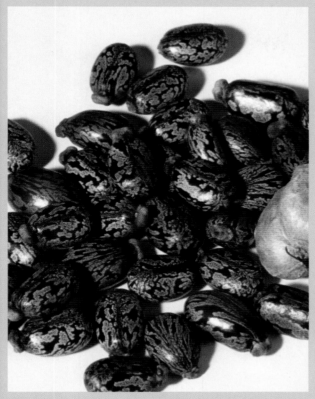

The beans of the castor tree have been used for their purgative properties for hundreds of years.

down the medical folklore and embraced millions of women patients. It is this folk medicine of rural communities which, blended with traditional lore of the American Indians in North America in the eighteenth and nineteenth centuries, produced the patent medicines peddled by traveling medicine men, snake doctors, and quacks.

Tainted by a reputation for superstition and quackery, coupled with the influence of advances in medical science presided over by eminent doctors such as Louis Pasteur, herbal practices were again pushed into obscurity in the nineteenth and twentieth centuries. But the end of the last century saw a renewal of interest in medical herbalism, its practitioners treating those who felt uneasy about the widespread use of drugs and their side-effects.

> *I consulted a private doctor last fall, desperate for a way to overcome hot flashes. Her remedies have been astonishingly successful. I take Menosan drops, a tincture made from the herb sage, three times every day plus one red clover tablet once daily. Supplements and a cream have eased a few other problems I have had in the past two to three years.*
>
> LINDA

Nowadays, you do not need to seek out the services of a "wise woman" for herbal remedies: You can buy them over the counter at health food outlets or through the Internet. On the other hand, you might choose to consult a well-qualified medical herbalist working in a resilient herbal market worth many millions of dollars a year. (A recent survey of the European herbal market valued the trade at 3.2 billion euro [3.4 billion American dollars].)

THE CONSULTATION

The herbalist will give you a thorough examination and will need details of your medical history and eating habits. Your blood pressure will be checked, and the practitioner will evaluate the overall balance of your body's systems—musculo-skeletal, nervous, cardiovascular, digestive, genito-urinary, and endocrine—to discover underlying and predisposing disharmonies.

It is you as a whole person who will be treated, not simply the complaint. Thus, entirely different remedies may be prescribed to two patients apparently suffering from the same problems.

You are unlikely to need frequent consultations unless you have a condition that requires close monitoring and

HERBS COMMONLY USED FOR PERIMENOPAUSAL AND MENOPAUSAL SYMPTOMS

Name of herb	For relief of	Recommendations
Balm	Tension, stress reactions, and depression	A tincture of 2–6 ml 3 times a day, or 2–3 teaspoons of dried herb steeped in 1 cup of boiling water twice a day
Black Cohosh	Hot flashes, anxiety, and depression	40-200 mg daily, use not to exceed six months
Chasteberry	Hot flashes	Prepared as a tincture, chastetree berry provides an average daily dose equal to 20 mg of the crude fruit or 30-40 mg of the fruit in a decoction
Gingko	Poor memory, mood swings, anxiety, and absent-mindedness	A daily dose of 120-160 mg of standardized gingko leaf extract
Ginseng	Fatigue, diminished work capacity, and loss of concentration	1 500 mg capsule can be taken 3–6 times a day. Use not to exceed three months
St John's wort	Depression	2-4 g of hypericin capsule, 1-2 times a day. The equivalent may be steeped in 1 cup of boiling water for 10 minutes to gain a similar amount
Valerian	Insomnia and tension	2–3 g, taken 1–3 times a day, is suggested as an anti-anxiety regimen

regular examinations. You can simply telephone the herbalist when you need more medicine, and any adjustments can be made, if necessary.

Many patients note a measurable degree of improvement within the first month of treatment, but one to two months of treatment for every year of illness may be required if the condition is chronic.

SAFETY

It is a persistent and popular misconception that herbal medicines are totally safe and free from side-effects. This is far from true, since many plants from which the remedies are made are known to be poisonous. Unfortunately, the full effects of toxic constituents of plants are difficult to assess. In the UK, herbal practitioners are permitted to use a few poisonous plants up to statutory maximum dosages. These substances are not permitted for general sale. Other countries have similar regulations, although there are no government standards on the quality of herbal products in the USA. Herbs can be labeled with information on effects on the body's structure and function, but must state that the FDA (Food and Drug Administration) has not reviewed them and they are not intended for use as drugs.

In 1978, Germany established Commission E to review the safety and use of over 1400 herbal drugs. The eight herbs in the table above were considered to be effective and safe for one or more perimenopausal or menopausal complaints.

HERBAL PREPARATIONS

Herbal medicines come in various forms, some of which are ready for use and some of which require preparation.

Many people choose to buy ready-made preparations, but others prefer to buy the raw materials and create their own remedies. Breaking down the herb samples to a suitable size used to be the hardest work of all the processes of preparation, entailing hours of labor with a pestle and mortar. Now, a kitchen blender will perform many functions quite adequately.

Water or a mixture of water and ethyl alcohol is usually added to the herbs. Sometimes acetic acid (vinegar), glycerol (or glycerine), and seed oils are used. A liquid that has the best chance of dissolving the required active ingredients is usually used. "Woody" material, such as bark and roots, has to be infused in hot water for a certain period.

Being natural products, herbal preparations are very variable in strength. The quantity of active ingredients differs widely from product to product. The raw material varies according to the climate and conditions in which it is grown, and the quality of the preparation will vary according to how it is treated and how many other ingredients are added. In addition, the dosage depends on how the herbs are prepared. For example, the longer teas are steeped, the stronger the dose.

COMBINING MEDICINES

Your medical herbalist will not advise you to stop taking drugs prescribed by your doctor but will usually work together with any orthodox treatment that may be deemed necessary. Many patients want to come off their prescribed drugs, and herbalists aim to reduce or eliminate the need for them.

FORMS OF HERBAL PREPARATION

Preparation	Description
Bulk herbs	*Raw, dried plant material in jars or bins; used in teas, tinctures; powdered for capsules, tablets*
Oils	*External use only, some are fatal if ingested; used in aromatherapy*
Tablets, capsules	*Stored and transported easily*
Teas	*Hot-water extracts, of which there are three types:*
	Beverages, teas, steeped for 1 to 2 minutes
	Infusions, steeped for 10 to 20 minutes
	Decoctions made of plant material simmered in boiling water for 10 to 20 minutes
Tinctures	*Alcohol extracts; highly concentrated; come in small bottles with eyedropper caps; few drops usually used*

SAFETY CONCERNS

Much of the concern about the safety, efficacy, and quality of herbal remedies may be removed following the European Union's traditional herbal medicines directive which came into force at the end of 2002. This will require manufacturers to register unlicensed products and produce them according to good pharmaceutical manufacturing practices.

BLACK COHOSH

At present, the most effective herbal medicine for treating menopausal symptoms is an extract of black cohosh (RemiFemin), which has been subjected to two clinical trials. The safety profile is positive with low toxicity, few and mild side-effects, and good tolerability. RemiFemin has been used in Germany since the 1950s.

SENSIBLE MEASURES

In general, herbal medicines may have a short-term role in managing the symptoms of menopause, but they are unlikely to be useful in treating the long-term aspects, particularly those related to osteoporosis. It is advisable to stop using any herbal remedy if, after a period of no more than several weeks, it is not clearly improving your condition. Most herbs do not take months to work; it is the condition that sets the pace. Always challenge a treatment if, after four weeks, you think the herbal remedy is not useful. If there are doubts, stop the medicine for a time and see if it is still necessary.·

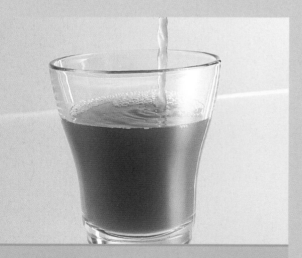

INFUSIONS

To make an infusion, use one teaspoon of dried herbs to one cup of boiling water; allow to infuse for 10 to 15 minutes, strain, and drink hot. Sweeten with honey if preferred.

DECOCTIONS

These are made from materials such as roots, barks, nuts, and seeds. Using the same proportion as for an infusion, place the mixture and water in a saucepan. Bring to the boil, then simmer for 10 minutes. Strain and drink hot.

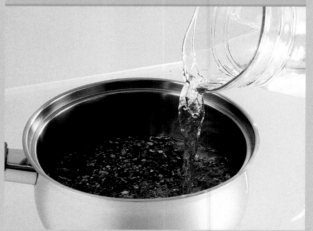

Homeopathy

Nearly 200 years ago, an eminent and conventionally qualified German physician published the first results of a form of treatment that he developed and used experimentally on himself and his family. His name was Samuel Hahnemann and he christened the principle of this treatment "homeopathy," from two Greek words—homios meaning "like" and pathos meaning "suffering."

In some ways, Hahnemann was a scientist but in others he was a metaphysician or even a mystic. He believed that life was sustained by a vital force and that disease was caused by some outside influence that disturbed the smooth functioning of the vital force, thus inducing symptoms of illness. His belief was that if you could discover and remove the cause of the trouble and stimulate the vital healing force of nature, then patients would heal themselves.

It had all begun when Hahnemann decided to see what would happen if he dosed himself with quinine, a remedy used to combat malaria. He was surprised to find that he developed a fever and other symptoms associated with malaria, even though he did not have the disease. These symptoms disappeared when he stopped taking the quinine. When he started taking quinine again, the symptoms recurred. Here was confirmation of Hippocrates' belief that if an individual who is suffering from an illness can be made to suffer symptoms similar to those produced by his illness, then he will be cured. The severity of symptoms and healing responses are dependent on the individual.

This "like cures like" principle forms the basis of homeopathy and is in stark contrast with conventional or "allopathic" medicine, which treats illness with an antidote rather than a similar substance. But this was not the only principle that distinguished Hahnemann's medical practice from that of his contemporaries.

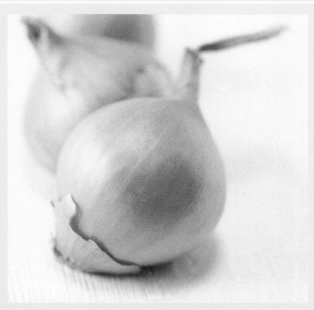

Onions are just one of the substances that are used for homeopathic remedies.

Dissatisfied with the medical practices of his day, which consisted mainly of "bleeding" and the use of large doses of dangerous drugs, he decided to dispense smaller doses of medicine. To his surprise, he found that the more the remedy was diluted, the more active it became.

Orthodox medicine was unimpressed. This paradox— that less of a substance could be more effective—was perhaps not surprisingly unacceptable to the scientific community of the time, as well as to modern skeptics who doubt the worth of giving extremely dilute solutions of dubious substances to the sick. Nevertheless, every year 4 percent of adults in the USA use a homeopathic medicine, while in the UK that figure is more than double that at 8.5 percent.

Hahnemann and his followers were ridiculed, yet they continued to experiment with all sorts of substances derived from minerals or animal and plant products, testing them in what he termed "provings." Over long periods his patients took small doses of various reputedly poisonous or medicinal substances, carefully noting the symptoms produced. Patients who were suffering from similar symptoms were then treated with these substances, with encouraging results.

An enormous amount of information was accumulated to form the main source of knowledge about homeopathy. By the time he died in 1843, Hahnemann had done provings on 99 substances. This increased to 600 more medicines by 1900, and today there are nearly 3,000 substances available to homeopaths. The materials include onion, Indian hemp, honey-bee sting venom, snake venom, and spiders, as well as sand, charcoal, common salt, and pencil lead. Hahnemann also advocated the use of single medicines rather than complex mixtures, reasoning that it was not possible to distinguish the effects of large numbers of drugs when they were mixed together.

There are two forms of homeopathy in use today: one which lays great emphasis on the use of highly dilute medicines and on certain philosophical, even semi-mystical ideas about disease and its causation, and a modern form based on fairly orthodox notions of pharmacology that largely ignores philosophical thought. But the essence of the homeopathic principle remains the same; it is the patient who is treated rather than the disease.

HOMEOPATHIC REMEDIES

A single remedy may be prescribed from a variety of sources and in a number of dilutions, such as pulsatilla (an anemone flower), sepia (a sea creature) or sulfur (a mineral). The homeopath has thousands of remedies to choose from, and the process of selecting the right one is individual. Just a handful of these remedies are readily available in pharmacies and health food shops, such as:

- Lachesis for poor memory, difficulty in concentrating, anxiety, and depression.

PUT TO THE TEST

A total of 657 patients received treatment for their pre- and postmenopausal complaints in a three-month study conducted in 1994 by 77 therapists in Germany.

Participants were given a combination homeopathic preparation consisting of agnus castus, black cohosh, ambergris, St. John's wort, common nettle, sepia, calcium, potassium, and gelsenium.

Two-thirds reported continuous and definite relief from their symptoms, and even though they did not achieve complete relief, they all said they intended to continue the treatment.

SERIOUS ILLNESS

Responsible homeopaths agree that many serious disorders—cancers, serious infections, etc.—do need treatment from orthodox practitioners.

- Pulsatilla for depression, weepiness, changeable moods, and headaches.
- Argentum nitricum and salvia for hot flashes.
- Graphites for irritability, difficulty in concentrating, depression, weepiness, and over-excitability.

However, it can be difficult to evaluate your own situation clearly, and consulting a homeopath for a professional opinion helps in finding the correct remedy in the right potency. This might be a lay practitioner (someone who may have had no formal training and possesses no accepted academic qualifications) or a doctor who is fully qualified through conventional medical training and who has undergone further training in homeopathy.

THE CONSULTATION

Your first homeopathy appointment may last as long as two hours, because making the correct diagnosis is a vitally important part of the treatment. You may be asked questions about the following:

- Your past health and life circumstances, the pattern of health in your family, your present condition
- What are the particular symptoms? What makes them worse or better—warmth, cold, eating, drinking, moving about, lying down, and so on?
- How do you feel about the condition? (Angry, resentful, depressed?)
- What are your underlying fears, moods, and anxieties?

Having gathered all the information needed and assuming that you do not need to be referred to a medical specialist, then the homeopath will analyze the answers you have supplied and formulate the appropriate medicine. This can then be obtained from your homeopathic pharmacist. Although they are completely different in their preparation and action, homeopathic medicines look much like any other medicines and are taken in the form of small pills, tablets, drops, granules, powders, and liquids.

SAFETY

Homeopathic remedies are completely safe, nontoxic, and nonaddictive.

COMBINING MEDICINES

It is perfectly safe to take antibiotics along with a homeopathic medicine, although the side-effects from the antibiotic may complicate the symptoms picture and thus make the choice of homeopathic treatment more difficult.

I consulted a registered homeopath who spent an hour-and-a-half asking me a number of questions about my general health, my current situation, major events in my life, and seemingly unrelated questions such as "How do you feel about frogs? And thunderstorms?" She reassured me that my symptoms of irritability, mood swings, change in sexual desire, irregular and heavy bleeding, random sweating, weight gain, sleeplessness, and palpitations were common when women were perimenopausal. Having listened carefully, she then prescribed a remedy—pulsatilla.

The first week I took it, I experienced violent mood swings and severe irritability to the point where I almost felt out of control. I had decided to give it one more week and then give up if there was no improvement. As if by magic, everything changed. I slept better, my periods became more regular, the bleeding lessened, my mood evened out, and I became altogether more pleasant to be with, both for my family and myself.

I would not hesitate to recommend homeopathy for this stage of a woman's life.

VICKI

A number of homeopathic substances have a very specific application in certain conditions, such as indigestion and bruising, and so they can successfully treat a large cross-section of the population. For instance, arnica ointment is very effective for healing bruises after an operation.

Some feeling of well-being is usually experienced within one week, even though the symptoms remain. However, if symptoms do not improve within two weeks of starting treatment, then a different medicine should be considered.

Stress—and how to live with it comfortably

Psychosocial factors—life stress situations, depression and social isolation—have been linked to increased risk of cardiovascular disease (pages 53 to 59). Whatever you do in your daily life and whatever your circumstances, you will encounter stress every day. It is part of the human condition begun even before birth. In fact, a baby can show signs of distress in its mother's womb. Stress is unavoidable, whether we are children or adults—single, divorced, married, or widowed.

Stress is a catalyst for change because it provides us with excitement, stimulation, and motivation. But it can accelerate to dangerous levels, and all of us need to learn ways of coping with stress.

- High levels of emotional stress increase susceptibility to illness.
- Chronic stress results in a suppression of our immune systems, which in turn increases our susceptibility to illness.
- Emotional stress also suppresses our immune systems and leads to hormonal imbalances.

It would be reassuring if at least our menopausal years were ones of contentment where a calmer, less frenetic pace replaced years of pressure. All too often this does not happen, usually because we allow ourselves to feel powerless in the face of the demands, needs, and expectations of other people, frequently as a consequence of our own lack of self-esteem.

In over 20 years work as a counselor, I have talked with hundreds of anxious midlife women about their stressful situations. One 52-year-old woman, Moira, initially described herself as being "on a roller-coaster of confusion," and her words are echoed by many of us when we cannot see "the wood for the trees." This happens when our lives are so crowded that we lose sight of our own selves.

Some women find that their brains are on the go all the time, and when this occurs it often leads to disturbed sleep patterns. Daily living is punctuated by erratic behavior that disrupts normal physical, mental, and spiritual functioning. If this strikes a chord with you, you need to know that you can help yourself. First you need to create a quiet half hour on your own with no interruptions so that you can:

- Identify where you are now.
- Reflect on and consider your options.
- Think about the elimination or better management of the stress in your life.

> *I was 48 years old and had come to a crossroads in my life: I'd worked part-time as an estate agent to help my daughters through university and now wanted to do something different. I had been doing yoga for 20 years and was encouraged to go on a teacher training course in the Bahamas. It was very tough, but I stuck with it and now teach three classes a week. I also teach a class at the local golf club and provide private classes in people's homes. My dream is to have a health food restaurant with a yoga center above it offering alternative therapies as well.*
>
> *I finally have a job that is more than merely a means to an end. I really enjoy the benefits I get from yoga and enjoy passing on those benefits to others.*
>
> **JANET**

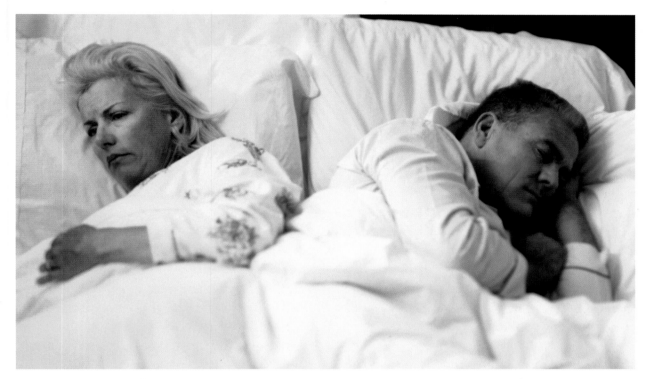

Sexual intimacy may be affected during the menopausal transition, and it will need patience and goodwill to re-establish.

From chaos to clarity

STEP 1

You will need a large pad of paper and a pen. Divide one sheet of paper roughly into four sections and write the following words at the top of each one:

> Where am I now?
> Where do I want to be?
> How am I going to get there?
> What is stopping me?

Complete the sections with the words and thoughts that come immediately to mind. This should take about five or six minutes.

By focusing on the here-and-now, you put yourself in center-stage, instead of the stressful situation. Maybe you have just drifted into your particular set of circumstances, with only a vague idea of what you were aiming for. Perhaps you have put your trust in fate. Now your concentrated effort can bring secret hopes and desires to the surface—and also allow expression of unhappy feelings.

There may not yet be total clarity, but certain words and phrases may well be thought-provoking. Perhaps you find yourself scribbling down other words and thoughts on another piece of paper. You have now begun the process of putting your particular roller-coaster into some sort of perspective.

STEP 2

The first step may have stirred up all manner of emotions for you, so this next one should be undertaken only when you feel ready for it.

Read through everything you have written down and highlight stressful issues that need special attention. Group them together under the following headings:

My personal relationships
My work outside my home

Select one of these and:

- Explore your options.
- Write down the possibilities for changes, even if some of them seem far-fetched.
- Formulate a plan of action.

If you are unsure about the best way forward, then a session with a counselor may help you to resolve your uncertainties.

You could also benefit from incorporating one or more of the activities and therapies covered on pages 90 to 103 into your life. Start by learning to relax properly using the exercises opposite.

Learning to relax

You may think—oh, that's easy! I relax every time I come home from work, kick off my shoes, and flop into a comfortable chair with my favorite drink. And yes, some of your tension falls away as you relax initially in a passive, unfocused way. But not all of it. Most of us have been conditioned to believe that we must constantly be active and productive, and our minds are likely to be preoccupied with all sorts of important issues.

Many of us assume that relaxation comes naturally to us, but it does not. Setting aside time for the two exercises opposite is a simple way to start really letting go. It may well feel a bit strange at first, but its effect can be both releasing and rejuvenating. These exercises can be practiced while lying in bed before falling asleep or at any time when you want to achieve really deep relaxation. They feature three distinctive elements:

- Focusing on particular muscles
- Creating tension by holding them
- Allowing relaxation

When you relax properly your entire body will be loose and totally at ease.

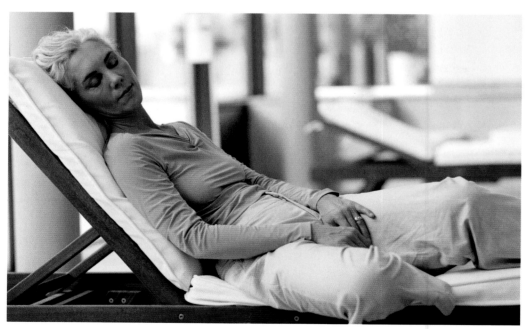

EXERCISE 1: A BREATHING SPACE

Your surroundings need to be warm and comfortable, and your clothes loose-fitting. If you try this exercise on the floor, use a soft cover, such as a large piece of foam rubber, a futon, or duvet.

1. Get into your chosen position and close your eyes.
2. Focus on your breathing; feel how the air goes in and out of your lungs.
3. Feel the weight and warmth of your body. As you relax deeper into yourself, you will feel even heavier as the warmth begins to envelop you.
4. Take a deep breath, expanding your diaphragm and ribs, hold it for two seconds, then sigh, releasing all the air from your lungs. Listen to the air as it is expelled. Repeat this five or six times.

From shoulder to shoulder

Hold each position to an even count of 5.

5. Hunch your shoulders as high as you can – hold them there – relax.
6. Tense the upper part of your arms – hold – relax.
7. Tense your complete arms – hold – relax.
8. Clench your fists – hold – relax.

On a lower level

9. Tense your buttocks – hold – relax. Do the same with your thighs and the calf muscles in your legs.
10. Draw your feet up in the direction of your upper body, as if you are straining to see them – hold – relax.
11. Curl your toes – hold – relax.

You are now fully relaxed and may drift off to sleep. Or you can return gradually to consciousness by counting down from 10 to 1.

EXERCISE 2: RELAXATION AND MENTAL IMAGERY

Mental imagery, also known as visualization, means forming an image in your mind, then creating a clear mental statement of what you want to happen. Some of us are more "visual" than others. Some people think primarily in images, others tend to sense or feel things, and some people think in words. You need to operate in the sense that is most natural to you in visualizing your desired outcome.

For example, if you have high blood pressure, you could visualize the problem as little muscles in the walls of your blood vessels tightening down, so that much higher pressure is needed for the blood to be driven through. Next, visualize the medication relaxing these little muscles in the blood vessels, your heart pumping evenly, with less resistance, and blood flowing smoothly through the vascular channels.

1. Set yourself a mental goal: for instance, the relief of repeated anxious feelings.
2. Prepare yourself with the relaxation exercises at left.
3. Retreat in your mind to a special place, perhaps a tropical beach. Allow yourself to use all your senses to explore it—to feel the warm sun, smell the plants, listen to the birds, feel the salt spray on your body, the sand tickling your toes.
4. When your special place is established, put yourself into the image to achieve your goal. A relaxed mind is receptive to anything you want to give it.
5. Make a positive mental statement about yourself, such as "I feel calm and in control."
6. Drift away gradually from your special place. When you open your eyes you will feel relaxed and refreshed. Do not get up quickly because the drop in blood pressure may make you feel light-headed.

Meditation

Meditation aims to achieve both relaxation of the body and a heightened state of awareness. Regular meditation can bring greater control over restless thoughts and emotions, leading to a sense of well-being. As a result, you will be able to shut yourself off from the world and find inner peace.

It is now generally accepted that our minds can influence mechanical bodily functions and the chemical balance that ensures good health. When our minds are persistently disturbed by unhappy thoughts and feelings, such as worry, anxiety and resentment, our energy levels are disrupted. These disruptions can cause physical symptoms of illness.

Meditation can offer considerable benefits. It has been found to be effective in:

- Regulating blood pressure.
- Stimulating blood circulation.
- Alleviating pain.
- Reducing muscular tension.
- Slowing down hormonal activity.

Although meditation is often associated with an ascetic, spiritual lifestyle, there is no need for you to renounce your own beliefs. It is enough to approach your meditation practice as just another element in your daily exercise routine. Take from it whatever you need—be it relief from stress, improved physical and mental health, or a sustained sense of well-being.

When you first start meditating, it is important to try to establish good habits, specifically those concerning correct posture and breath control. Both of these are useful in aiding your concentration when your thoughts wander.

POSTURE

Although the various postures described and illustrated on these pages are interchangeable, you could attempt all of them initially, persevering with each for a week until settling with one or two that suit you.

Lying down

If you choose to lie down on your back, make sure you support your neck with a cushion. Let your arms hang loosely by your side and keep your legs straight. Do not cross your legs or put your hands on your body.

Sitting

Choose a straight-backed chair to sit in so that you get support and do not cramp your diaphragm. Your feet

This is a comfortable position to relax in. Simply kneel on the floor, place a cushion behind your knees and sit down.

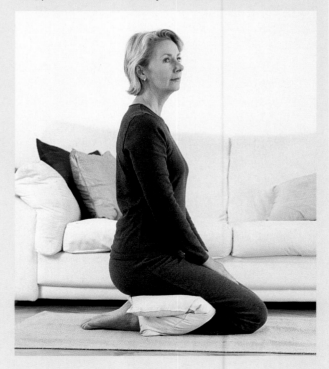

should be flat on the floor and slightly apart in line with your shoulders. Place your hands on your knees, palms down—or up, if you prefer a symbolic gesture of openness.

Classical postures

The traditional cross-legged postures that are used in yoga require a degree of suppleness you may not possess. An alternative to the classical postures is to rest on your heels with a cushion supporting your buttocks, as in the Japanese tradition.

STARTING TO MEDITATE

When you first learn to meditate, the most difficult aspect is the quieting of the mind. Initially, you will probably find lots of other things that seem in more urgent need of your attention, and you may be tempted to put off your meditation indefinitely.

It is important to begin with simple exercises to establish good practice. This basic candle gazing meditation will help you to establish the habit of sitting still in silence and will train your mind to focus on the object of the exercise. Practice it twice a day for six days, then rest for one day before moving on to the other meditations described on page 92.

Candle gazing

1. Place a candle in front of you so that the candle is in line with the point between your eyebrows.
2. Now gaze at the candle and observe the flicker, the candle's size, and every aspect of it.
3. After 30 to 60 seconds, close your eyes and keep the flame as steady as you can. At first, the afterglow will fade and you will be left with nothing. You then need to open your eyes and repeat the

process. Eventually, you will retain an optical image of the candle and the flicker of light in your mind.

4. When the flicker of light starts to disappear, force the image to stay. This trains your mind to concentrate. At first it will seem impossible to maintain the image, but with continued practice it becomes easy.
5. Focus your attention on one thought, and keep breathing deeply while concentrating on that thought.
6. Become one with the flame so that there is no space between it and you. Enjoy the sense of spaciousness and expansion.
7. When you feel ready, slowly come back to waking consciousness and open your eyes.

Learn to meditate by training your mind to focus on the flickering flame of a candle.

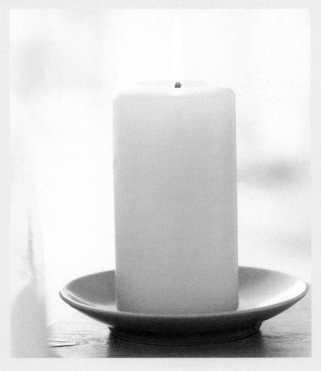

OTHER MEDITATIONS

Helpful meditations in your present circumstances could include the following:

Pain reduction

If you suffer from headaches or other pains, you may find meditation useful. A pain-reduction method involves imagining what your pain looks like.

1. Prepare yourself with the relaxation exercises on page 89.
2. Focus on your pain. What color is it? See its color, shape, and size clearly. It may be a red ball. It may be the size of a tennis ball or a grapefruit.
3. Mentally project the ball out into space, maybe two yards away from your body.
4. Make the ball bigger, about the size of a football, then shrink it to the size of a pea. Now let it become whatever size it chooses to be.
5. Begin to change the ball's color; make it pink, then light green.
6. Now take the green ball and put it back where you originally saw it. At this point, notice whether or not your pain has decreased.

Getting rid of an upset

1. Get into your chosen relaxed position.
2. Close your eyes and breathe naturally. When you feel suitably relaxed, imagine that you are sitting at a desk. In front of you are pen, paper, envelope, candle, matches, and a bowl filled with water.
3. Look down at the blank paper in front of you and take up the pen.
4. Now write a letter to the person who you believe has upset you, describing your feelings and explaining the situation as you understand it. It is necessary to express your feelings, because the primary purpose of this exercise is to face and free your emotions. Once you have released your anger, you will hopefully see the situation from a less impassioned perspective. Having done so, you may feel able to forgive and forget.
5. When you have finished your letter, imagine addressing the envelope and putting the letter inside.
6. Visualize lighting the candle. Hold the envelope over the flame, and when it has curled into ashes, drop it into the bowl.
7. When you feel ready, slowly come back to waking consciousness and open your eyes.

Relationship problems

It takes two to create difficulties in any relationship, and it can be very hard to break the "blaming" habit.

1. Get into your chosen position.
2. Close your eyes, breathe naturally, and when you feel suitably relaxed, visualize the other person.
3. Soften your heart by meditating on compassion.
4. See the other person as a being whose human nature is as fallible as your own.
5. Draw the person toward you and embrace him or her, while repeating the following affirmation: "You and I are enjoying a good, positive relationship. Energy is flowing freely between us." Then release the person and watch as he or she fades into the distance.

Tension will be diffused, and you will be able to talk matters through calmly.

Writing a letter may help you to release your anger.

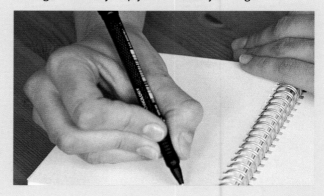

Yoga

Yoga is often seen as a mystical Eastern relaxation system that involves intricate postures that only the most supple and double-jointed of us would dare to attempt. But as many people have discovered, the movements can be very simple and beneficial whether you are 9 or 90 years old, even if your joints are creaking or you are ill or disabled.

Some 4,000 years ago in ancient India, the original practitioners were philosophers or yogis who lived as hermits. Today, the benefits of yoga have spread internationally and it is now practiced in nonreligious, noncultural-based classes all over the Western world, from local adult education classes to centers and organizations devoted exclusively to yoga. This ancient way to better health has been adopted by people of all ages and from all walks of life.

Most classes are based on hatha yoga or physical yoga. "Ha" means the sun, which represents masculine energy, and "Tha" means the moon, representing feminine energy.

BASIC UNDERSTANDINGS

The three principles of hatha yoga are:
- Pranayama (breathing). This breathing technique encourages us to make full use of our lungs, balances the masculine and feminine energies within our bodies, and boosts energy levels.
- Asanas (postures). These are held for as long as possible to build stamina as well as alter the energy in our bodies.
- Dhyana (meditation).

Stretching is the best way to achieve head-to-toe fitness and reduce stress in muscles. In yoga exercise, stretching is an integral part of each movement. Cats are a wonderful example of stretching, and their suppleness is second to none in the animal kingdom.

Yoga is a gentle exercise system that is believed to encourage union of your body, mind, and spirit and to restore balance in the following ways: It relaxes your muscles and improves suppleness, fitness, and physical function. It relaxes your mind and shows you how to control stress and destructive emotions. It needs to be practiced regularly to have a lasting effect, and is usually taught in classes lasting from one to two hours.

WHAT HAPPENS IN A CLASS?

Classes vary in structure, but in a 90-minute class you would usually begin by focusing on breath control for about 10 minutes, followed by 15 to 20 minutes of gentle warm-up exercises. It takes time to master the postures. The teacher will reassure you about your level of achievement and encourage you not to push yourself too hard. Postures are usually performed for about 25 minutes, followed by 20 minutes of relaxation exercises. The class may end with 5 to 10 minutes of reflection and advice to practice at home in a warm, quiet, and well-ventilated room.

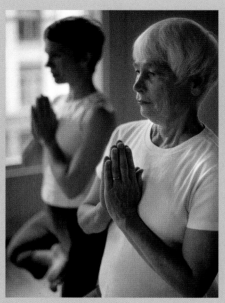

Yoga postures are usually performed for about 25 minutes in a class, followed by 20 minutes of relaxation.

Massage

Three thousand years ago, the wealthy citizens of Greece and Rome began every day with an experience called "the bath." For several hours in the early morning they devoted themselves to body care. They either bathed themselves or were bathed by attendants. Intricate exercise programs were developed to strengthen their bodies, while especially stiff muscles were rubbed with warm oils. A full body massage under the hands of skillful slaves awoke the nerves, stimulated the sluggish blood, and freed the action of the joints. Finally, the entire body was rubbed with a fine oil to keep the skin elastic and supple all through the day.

The two-hour morning bath has been replaced in our advanced civilization with a five-minute experience called the shower. This is a pity because, on its most basic level, massage is therapeutic simply because it is an intensely pleasurable experience. The desire to touch and be touched is one of our strongest instincts: We touch each other to show love, to offer security, and to feel good. We can exist without many things, but physical contact is not one of them.

Apart from the brain, the skin is the body's most complex organ. Each square centimeter of it contains hundreds of receptors sensitive to touch, pain, pressure, heat, and cold.

The basis of modern massage was developed by a Swedish gymnast turned therapist called Professor Per Henrik Ling (1776–1839). He formulated the principles of what became known as Swedish massage.

Today, massage can be found in therapy rooms, beauty salons, homes, sports clubs, and hospitals.

THE CONSULTATION

Your first appointment normally begins with the therapist writing down details about:

- Why you have come.
- Your current state of health.
- Your medical history.
- Details of any medication you take.
- General lifestyle inquiries.

You will be asked to undress, normally in privacy, and to lie on the massage table. You will not have to undress completely, if you prefer not to. But even if you do strip completely, the therapist will cover you with a towel and only uncover the parts of the body on which she or he needs to work.

The therapist might massage your back, work down your body, then ask you to turn over and work down your front, paying particular attention to knotty or tense areas. The massage should be relaxing, although you may feel pain in tense areas. You should not feel severe pain, so speak up if this happens.

A full body massage can last 90 minutes but is usually an hour. Everyone reacts differently to the treatment: You may feel relaxed, energized, slightly tired, or ache a little the next day. You might cry during the session. This is not unusual if you have been bottling up feelings.

A massage can help you to feel relaxed.

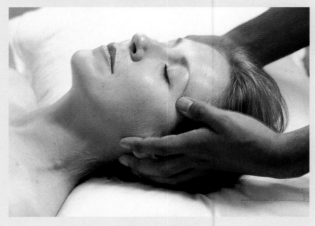

massage for menopause

There are trigger points within the abdominal wall that, when treated, can bring relief to menopausal symptoms. Here is a massage you can ask a friend or partner to do.

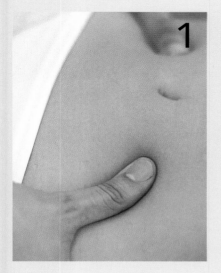

1 Place the pads of your thumbs about 3 inches (7 cm) on either side of the navel and, using your body weight, lean in toward the navel and hold for five seconds. Repeat two or three times.

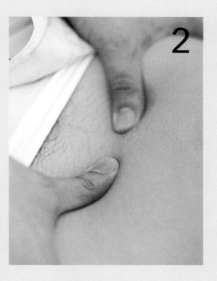

2 Move your thumbs close together and, using the pads, work as in step 1 downward in a straight line, from just below the navel to end level with the hips. Then work back up, finishing with your thumbs about 3 inches (7 cm) on either side of the navel.

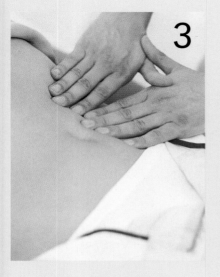

3 Using very light strokes and your hands relaxed and close together, place them on the mid-abdomen, level with the navel, and stroke gently toward the groin and return. Make sure that you massage both sides of the abdomen equally.

WHAT DIFFERENCE COULD MASSAGE MAKE TO MY STRESSFUL LIFE?

Basic massage techniques, such as stroking, kneading, wringing, pummelling, and knuckling, will stimulate your physical and emotional release in two ways—by a mechanical and a reflex action.

The mechanical effects of massage

The mechanical effects are the physical results of pressing, squeezing, and moving the soft tissue. This can be either relaxing or stimulating. For instance, your muscular tension can cause sluggish circulation because it forces your body's blood vessels to constrict.

Massaging the muscles frees up such tension and stimulates the circulation so blood flows freely, carrying oxygen and nutrients to where they are needed. It can help to normalize blood pressure, easing the pressure on arteries and veins.

Massage also stimulates the lymphatic system, encouraging it to carry waste products out of the body and defending it against infection.

The reflex action

The reflex action is an involuntary response of one part of your body to the stimulation of another. Because your body, mind, and emotions form one intricate organism connected by energy channels and a complex nervous system with receptors in the skin, stimulus in one part of your body can affect several other parts. For example, a relaxing back massage can also ease leg pain.

The four stages of healing

There are four stages in the healing process:

1. *Relief*
   The first few treatment sessions will relieve your pain, reduce tension and sedate stressed nerves.

They may not necessarily solve your problems, but massage alleviates the symptoms so that you feel better.

2. *Correction*
   The therapist can now work on the underlying cause to prevent the return of the problem. Correctional work could include retuning muscles, decongesting a sluggish lymph system, or freeing up muscle fibers that are knotted or scarred.

3. *Strengthening*
   This is important if you have a badly damaged area. Massage can strengthen the surrounding tissues, enabling them to provide adequate support when your injury has healed.

4. *Maintenance*
   Your therapist may recommend a regular check-up, much as dentists do.

THE POWER OF MASSAGE

In 1990, a study was carried out on 30 surgical patients at St. Mary's Hospital, London, in connection with pain relief and insomnia. The patients were massaged on the back, face, or feet and were then monitored for any physical or psychological changes. Most reported relief from pain, anxiety, and muscle spasm, as well as improved sleep and general well-being. The two nurses who performed the massage also reported a better rapport with their patients.

Reflexology

Feet and hands, two hard-working parts of the body, have always been popular sites for massage. The origins of reflexology evidently reach back to ancient Egypt as evidenced by a wall carving in the tomb of the renowned doctor Ankmahor, which shows doctors working on their patients' hands and feet. The accompanying hieroglyphics translate as the patient saying "Don't do anything that hurts" and the doctor replying "I shall act so you praise me," which can be seen as confirmation that this scene depicts a medical technique and not a beauty treatment.

To give a reflexology treatment, a therapist mainly uses her thumb, or sometimes her finger, to apply pressure to different points to release any blockage.

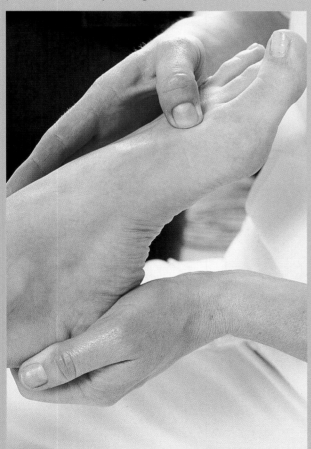

Doctors in Japan, India, and China developed their own methods of foot therapy, and this knowledge of Eastern therapies may have been brought to the West by adventurers such as Marco Polo who wrote that he much admired the Chinese health system.

Reflexology as we know it today was developed in the twentieth century by an American doctor, William Fitzgerald, an ear, nose and throat specialist at Boston General Hospital. He used the principles enshrined in zone therapy, in which the body is divided into ten vertical zones running from the tips of the toes to the top of the head and back down to the fingertips. All the parts of the body within one zone are linked. By applying pressure to one part of the body, Dr. Fitzgerald was delighted to find it was possible to relieve pain in other areas within the same zone.

Nowadays, zone therapy relies solely on the zones to determine the area to be worked, whereas reflexology takes the zones as well as the anatomical model to determine the area or areas to be worked.

THE CONSULTATION

Your first appointment will probably last for about 90 minutes, and you will be asked about yourself and why you have come for treatment.

- Details of your medical history will be needed, including childhood illnesses, accidents, or operations.
- You need to tell the therapist if you are under the care of a doctor or receiving drug treatment for any illness or any chronic (long-term) condition.
- You will be asked how you feel about yourself and your life—your work and leisure activities, as well as your eating, drinking, and lifestyle habits.

You will be asked to remove your shoes and socks or tights and to sit down in a reclining chair or lie on a treatment couch. Your feet may be wiped with some cotton soaked in witch hazel, followed by an application of either cream or talcum powder, which makes it easier to carry out the treatment.

Before giving attention to any problem areas, first one foot, and then the other, will be worked on. Pressure is applied to various points on them. If you feel pain or tenderness in any area, this is an indication of a blockage or imbalance in the corresponding organ or body part. The intention is not to cause you pain, but pain is a sign of blocked energy. This can be indicated by crystalline deposits under the skin, which can feel like grains of sugar, or the reflexes can be taut or particularly spongy.

If you are relaxing in a chair, you will be able to watch the techniques used by the reflexologist. These may include the following:

- *Thumb walking.* This is done with the pad of the thumb, which is pressed into the reflex points. After a few seconds, some of the pressure is released, the thumb slides along (like a caterpillar), stops, and presses again.
- *Finger walking.* This is similar to thumb walking, except that it is done with the side of the index finger, and using the thumb and other three fingers for support.
- *Rotating.* The thumb is pressed and rotated into the reflex point.
- *Flexing.* The toes are held in one hand while pressure is applied with the thumb of the other hand. The foot is then bent gently backward and forward, so that the thumb presses and releases the point in a rhythmic fashion.

No one knows exactly how reflexology works beyond the physical act of stimulating nerve endings in the feet. We know that there are 70,000 of these nerve endings on the sole of each foot that, when stimulated, can send messages along the pathways of the autonomic nervous system to all areas of the body and brain. By applying pressure to a particular point, known as a reflex point or area, the therapist can stimulate or rebalance the energy in the related zone. For example, your left kidney, which is in zone 2 of the left side of your body, is reflected at the same point in zone 2 of the left foot. If you have a problem in your left kidney, you might develop problems in your left eye, because the eyes and kidneys are both linked by the energy in zone 2.

CAN IT HELP MY HOT FLASHES?

Reflexology works well for any conditions that need to be cleared or regulated, such as menstrual irregularities, stress, fatigue, and aches and pains. If you consult a reflexologist for menopausal symptoms, it is likely that your feet will be worked all over, with special attention paid to the endocrine glands. The therapist will end by pressing the solar reflex on both feet.

PROVING A POINT

In a randomized controlled study in the USA undertaken in1993, ear, hand, or foot reflexology or a placebo treatment (treating inappropriate reflex zones, too roughly or too lightly) was given to 35 women suffering from PMS. Each woman kept a symptom diary for two months before, during, and after eight half-hour reflexology treatments. Thirty-nine symptoms were assessed on a four-point scale. The women given reflexology treatments showed a 46 percent reduction in the PMS symptoms and discomfort. The placebo group had only a 25 percent reduction.

reflexology for menopause

A reflexology treatment can work wonders. It benefits your body's systems and also provides the relaxing benefits of a foot massage. This sequence works on the reproductive and endocrine systems, including the thyroid, to help you through the transition.

1 First, find the thyroid reflex point, located on the top of the foot at the base of the big toe. Using your index finger, hook in and press this point for 5 seconds.

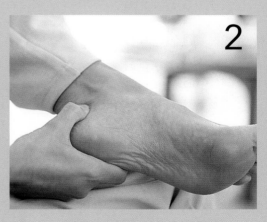

2 Next, gently work your foot in the area between the back of the heel and the ankle bone. Gently walk all four fingers up to the ankle bone. Find the ovary point and press for a count of 5 seconds.

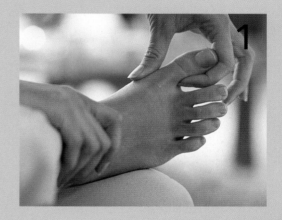

Aromatherapy

If you have enjoyed a full body massage, then your pleasure may be enhanced by the addition of essential oils used by practitioners of aromatherapy. These oils are aromatic essences extracted from plants, flowers, trees, fruit, bark, grasses, and seeds. About 150 essential oils have been extracted, each with its own unique scent and healing properties.

All essential oils contain antiseptic properties: some have particular ones that make them antiviral, anti-inflammatory, pain-relieving, or antidepressant. Others are stimulating, relaxing, aid digestion, or have diuretic properties.

Research indicates that the scent of essential oils can exert specific therapeutic effects on our minds and emotions. The oil molecules are so small that they can be absorbed through the pores of the skin, affecting the skin itself, the bloodstream, and the whole body, including the brain. Heat also helps their absorption, either through warm hands in a massage or from hot bath water.

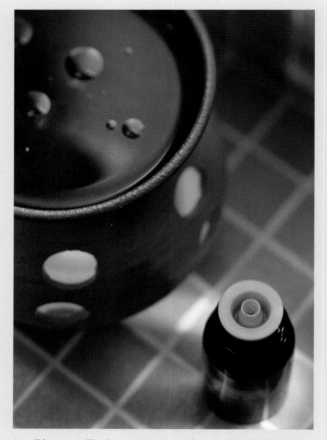

An oil burner will release the scent of essential oils into the air, providing natural fragrance, while distributing their therapeutic benefits.

THE CONSULTATION

Your first appointment with an aromatherapist will last between one and one-and-a-half hours. As with all forms of holistic therapy, the therapist will need to know:

- About you, your medical history, and why you have come.
- Which oils would be best to use, but also ones which should be avoided. Some oils are not safe to use if you have blood pressure problems, are epileptic, or have had a recent operation.
- If you are taking any medicines or homeopathic remedies. Strong smells can negate the effects of the latter.
- What mood you are in and what kind of day you have had.

You will be asked to undress and lie down on the massage table with a towel over you. (You need not undress completely if you feel uncomfortable doing so.)

The therapist will leave the towel over you and move it as he or she works around your body. That way you can stay warm and also feel less exposed.

The aromatherapist might decide on a blend of oils thought to suit you, or you may be asked if there are any oils you especially like. Then, with this blend of oils, the therapist will begin your massage, which lasts about 30 to 45 minutes.

The combination of touch and the therapeutic benefits of the oils improves circulation and releases trapped energy from the muscles. The fragrance also promotes feelings of well-being. For maximum benefit, you may be asked not to bathe or shower for a few hours after the massage so that the oils are absorbed throroughly and completely.

Once they have done their work, the oils will leave your body in various ways: Some are exhaled or excreted in urine and feces, while others are removed through perspiration. The process can take up to six hours in a healthy person but up to 14 hours in someone who is unhealthy or seriously overweight.

ESSENTIAL OILS FOR MENOPAUSE

Bergamot is excellent for anxiety, depression, and stress. It is a cleansing tonic for the uterus.

Cypress has a calming effect on the mind, soothing anger and frustration.

Clary sage can be used for menstrual problems, depression, and anxiety.

Fennel is good for menopausal problems, such as irregular periods, premenstrual tension, and low sexual response.

Geranium is useful for PMS, menopause, and anxiety.

Lavender is good for insomnia and headaches.

You can use aromatherapy solutions at home, too.

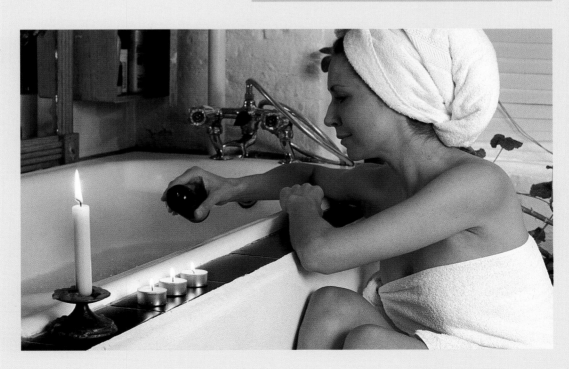

Getting away from it all

Many women in their menopausal years feel as though they are swept along by a tide of events beyond their control without a chance for a little peaceful living. Our lives are filled with preoccupations, distractions, and responsibilities, and however much we may yearn for peace, there seems little chance of making the time and space for it.

Going on a retreat is a deliberate attempt to step outside ordinary life, and to create a place and time of peace and quiet where distractions are at a minimum. Here is a space for you to contemplate the deepest feelings and thoughts about yourself and your relationships. Because everything we feel and do is filtered through our sense of self—call it self-awareness, self-identity, or consciousness—this sense is intrinsic to being human.

As you search for your true self, you may find a surprising void—an empty inner space you never knew existed. Suddenly there are no friends, children, partners, pets, television, work, or the constant background of human activity. There is no gossip, no grumbling, no meetings, no decisions, no interference. You are faced with you alone. You begin to slip into a slower physical, menta,l and emotional gear and start to think differently. Taking stock is what going on a retreat is all about.

WHO GOES ON RETREATS?

People of all ages and from all walks of life take advantage of the benefits of going on retreat—students, homemakers, grandparents, businessmen and women, millionaire celebrities, and the unknown poor. Men and women of all faiths and those of none go on retreat.

You will find many different types of retreat advertised in magazines and on the Internet. Most aim towards self-discovery of an experiential nature, and they can vary in duration from a single day to a week or longer.

- **Day retreats** These can be very flexible. It might be a day for silence, a day based on a theme, or an activity-centered day—time for group discussion, talks, or lessons given in meditation technique.

- **Weekend retreats** These are often run along the following lines: You arrive on Friday evening and, after settling your things in your room, meet the retreat leader and other guests. After supper you meet for a short talk about the weekend and are given a timetable. From that time on, you cease talking unless it is to the retreat leader or during a group discussion or shared prayer. There will be time for walks, reading, and just resting—simple, easy, and peaceful.

- **Healing retreats** These may use prayer, meditation, chanting, or the laying-on of hands.

Going on retreat means that you will have lots of time for reading, resting and quiet contemplation.

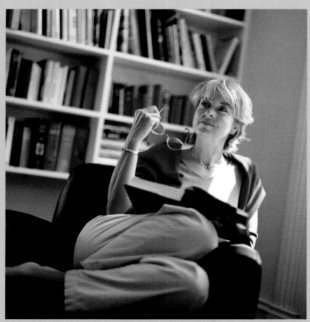

Healing may be concerned with a physical complaint or with healing the whole person in order to eliminate obstacles to personal and spiritual growth.

- **Lesbian retreats** These often have themes that bear directly on living as a lesbian within society and that link into spiritual matters.

- **Private retreats** In these you go alone as an individual. It is usually a silent time in which you find solitude in order to reflect, rest, and meditate. In many monasteries and retreat houses, you may arrange to take your meals in your room or separately from others so that you can maintain this framework of silence.

- **Embroidery, calligraphy, and painting retreats** Themed retreats focus on awakening personal creativity through a craft or art form. There are many other themes, such as pottery, poetry, music, or gardening.

Having placed yourself among strangers, you may meet people you like at once, those you do not want to know better, and those who make a nuisance of themselves—the sort of person who has some problem and cannot help talking about it to all and sundry. Equally, you may encounter those who are certain their beliefs hold the key to life. If you do not want to listen to them, you can walk away. Alternatively, you might find it both charitable and instructive to really listen to what the person is saying, even if you do not believe a word of it. And you do not have to discuss any of your beliefs or feelings unless you want to do so.

Going on retreat is about refreshing yourself, relaxing, and taking a journey into your deeper self. Reassessment of

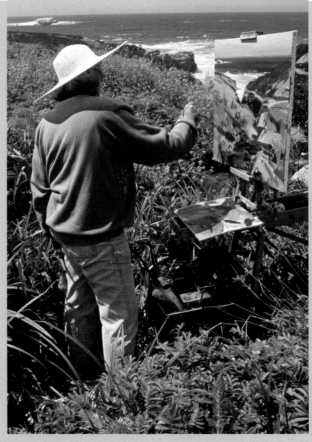

If you enjoy a craft, such as painting, then a retreat that allows you to focus on your creativity might suit you.

your life, relationships, and values can guide you into the future. If the opportunity is there, why not take advantage of it? It may prove to be an important pathway to better health.

BEFORE YOU BOOK...
If you have a disability, you will need to double-check the facilities before booking because many retreat centers and guest accommodations have not yet been updated to the standard set for the disabled.

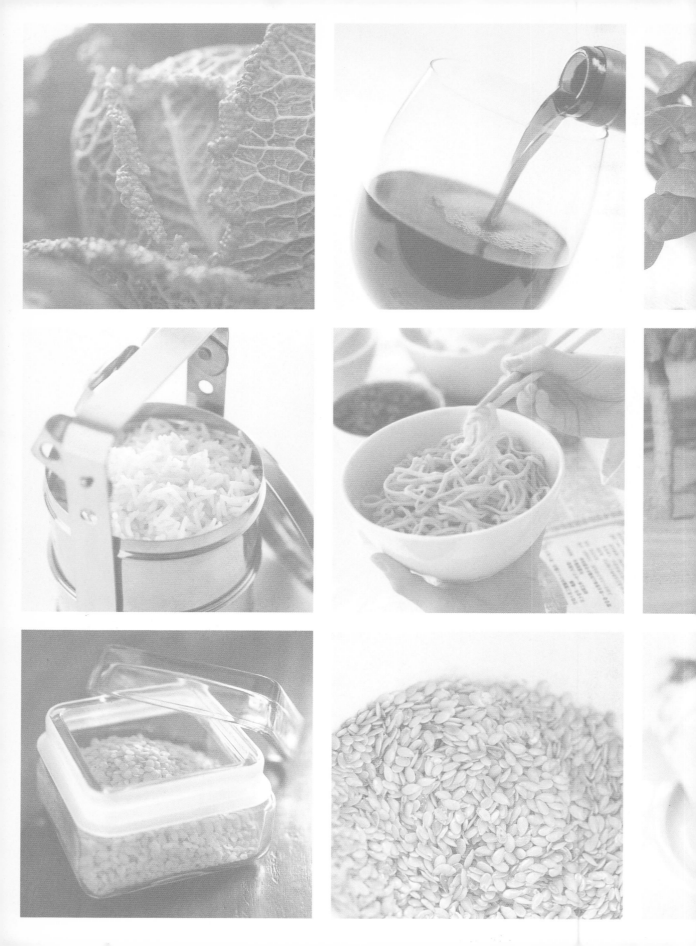

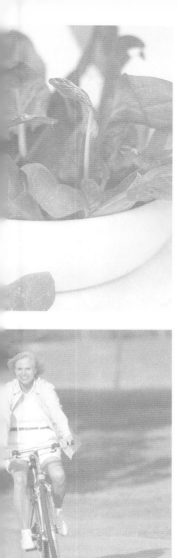

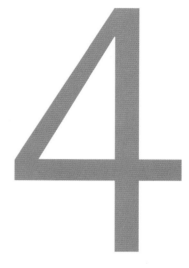

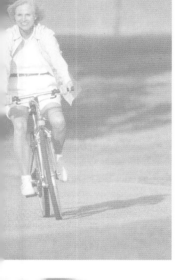

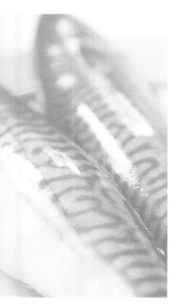

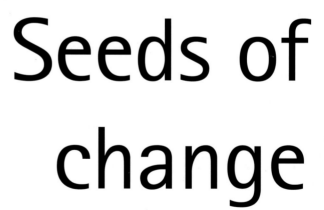

Seeds of change

Your diet and the menopause

The previous two chapters have demonstrated the variety of options open to you when considering HRT and its natural alternatives.

You may be convinced by the women who have spoken about their zest for living, happier feelings, and renewed energy levels when taking HRT, both for menopausal symptoms and as a long-term therapy. This is what you want for yourself. The simplicity of this treatment is especially appealing as you juggle the work and personal elements of a busy life. But you have also given more thought to these pressures, and realize you run a real risk of burnout unless you take time out for yourself.

Perhaps you are booked into a hospital for a hysterectomy and oophorectomy (removal of ovaries), and you are unable to take HRT afterward because of your family history of breast cancer. Your doctor has strongly

emphasized the need for low-dosage HRT post-operatively, and that regular mammograms will monitor your situation. You now realize there is a possible option in taking the SERM raloxifene (see page 49) and perhaps combining it with progesterone cream to counteract the abrupt loss of important hormones after the operation. An herbal or homeopathic remedy may be an option if your menopausal symptoms resurface.

On the other hand, you may be delighted to find that relief of your menopausal symptoms is possible through herbal or homeopathic remedies. You may consider HRT unnecessary for this transitory stage in your life. If your vagina is sore and painful during sexual intimacy, you can discuss this with your doctor and ask for a prescription for a vaginal ring.

However, there is another important consideration that affects all of us, whatever our ages. It is what might be termed "food fitness," and in this chapter we shall explore what this means.

Cycling can be fun when away from crowded cities, and is excellent exercise, whatever your age.

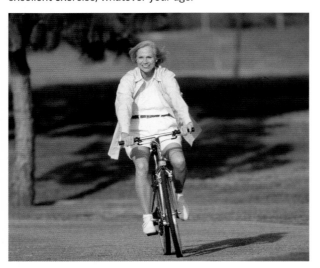

A question of balance

Perhaps you think you have maintained a healthy eating lifestyle while cooking for your family, but you are alarmed to discover that a dress you bought a couple of years ago doesn't fit. Can this be middle-age spread?

Taking stock of your eating and drinking habits *now* will stand you in good stead for the rest of your life. This does not mean giving up food and drink you enjoy, rather

"Tell me what you eat: I will tell you what you are." *(Jean-Anthelme Brillat-Savarin, 1825)*

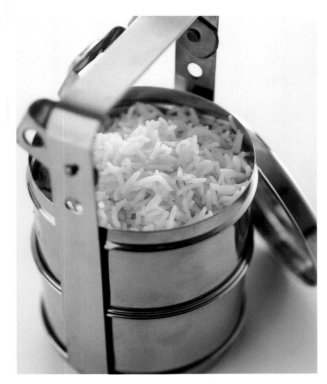
Using a steamer to cook food preserves all the vitamins which are often lost in conventional cooking.

recognizing how you can benefit by introducing exciting new perspectives to it and modifying some of the less helpful aspects.

As a child some 60 years ago, I ate and drank basic, nutritious, wholesome—and predictable—food. I recall wholegrain bread, meat and two vegetables, rice pudding, and lots of milk. Today, the impact of foreign trade and travel is reflected in the food we buy: pizzas, curries, and rice, as well as a vast array of pastas, sauces, cereals, cheeses, fish, meat, and exotic fruits and vegetables. All stimulate our taste buds and empty our wallets. Theoretically, Western society is now better fed than ever before. The reality is that many of us live in a "toxic food environment" of cheap fatty food, pervasive food advertising, and sedentary lives.

However self-assured and confident we are about our food choices, almost every week dire warnings appear in the media about the dangers of meat, coffee, chocolate, butter, etc. Yet, contradictory statements extolling their virtues are as likely to hit the headlines in the future. So how do we sort out fact from fiction?

Back to basics

Your body needs nutrients to maintain your physical, mental, and emotional well-being. The process began when you were a fetus in your mother's womb. As you developed from babyhood, essential nutrients determined your growth. Basically, your food is made up of the following three elements:

- Carbohydrates
- Protein
- Fats

CARBOHYDRATES

Carbohydrates are your body's main source of energy for all its functions. They are found in all vegetables, fruits, starches, and grains and, in its purest form, in refined sugar.

There are two types of carbohydrates—complex and simple. Complex carbohydrates give a slow release of energy because it takes time for our digestive tracts to break them down into the simplest substances that our bodies can use. Simple carbohydrates are best avoided where possible: They make your blood sugar rise steeply as a lot of sugar is pumped quickly into your system, then drop quickly as the sugar is rapidly burned. After a couple of hours, your energy levels plummet and you feel hungry again.

Complex carbohydrates

- Grains—wheat, rye, oats, rice, barley, and corn
- Beans—lentils, kidney beans, chickpeas, etc.
- Vegetables
- Fiber in grains, beans, and vegetables

Simple carbohydrates

- Fruit, honey, white and brown sugar, and glucose in high-energy drinks

You may be surprised to see fruit described as a simple carbohydrate. Fruit (and honey) contain fructose (also called fruit sugar), which is a simple sugar. However, the fiber content of the fruit is a complex carbohydrate, that slows the digestion rate. Fructose is fine when taken in whole fruits, like apples and pears, but not when used in the refined form of powdered white fructose.

PROTEINS

Proteins are found in their largest concentrations in animal foods such as meat, fish, poultry, eggs and cheese, vegetables, foods such as nuts and seeds, and in high-protein legumes, such as beans.

FATS

There is more confusion about dietary fat than almost anything else. It is seen as the villain of our eating habits, responsible for weight gain and its ensuing sluggish metabolism. We have all read about low-fat diets and

PROSTAGLANDINS

Beneficial prostaglandins (hormone-like regulating substances) are made by our bodies from omega 3 oils. These prostaglandins are particularly useful at the time of menopause because they help lower blood pressure and decrease sodium (salt) and water retention.

no-fat diets. Indeed, many of us have tried them. Sorting out fact from fiction about the nature of fats can help you determine how much you should increase or decrease it in your food fitness plan.

Basically, there are two types of fat—saturated and unsaturated:

Saturated fat

This is found in meat, dairy products, such as cheese, ice cream, milk, and tropical oils, like palm kernel oil and coconut oil. If you eat too many foods full of saturated fats, they will do their best to lay themselves down as fat stores. Hence the connection between fat intake and hardening of the arteries (see page 54).

Olives and olive oil are an excellent source of omega 3 essential fatty acids.

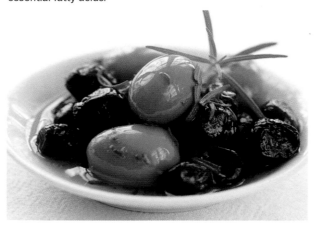

Oily fish, such as mackerel, contain oils that can help prevent the onset of heart disease.

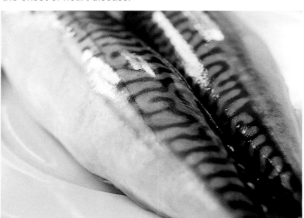

EVENING PRIMROSE AND HOT FLASHES

A randomized, double-blind, placebo-controlled study to evaluate the efficacy of evening primrose oil was set up for six months in 1994. It involved 56 menopausal women all of whom were suffering hot flashes at least three times a day. Half of them took four capsules of evening primrose oil twice a day. Analysis of diaries kept by the women showed it had no benefit over placebo in the alleviation of menopausal flashing, other than a reduction in the maximum number of night sweats.

Unsaturated fat

This is a group of fats that includes the essential fatty acids (EFAs), which are essential for our health. EFAs are a vital component of every human cell, and our bodies need them to insulate our nerve cells, keep our skin and arteries supple, balance our hormones, and keep us warm.

Unsaturated fat comes in two forms: monounsaturates, such as olive oil, and polyunsaturates, found in corn, sunflower seeds, and peanuts. Within this group there is a further division into:

Omega 3 fatty acids

The most important of these is alpha-linolenic acid, found in fish oils and flaxseed oil, walnuts, pumpkin seeds, and dark green vegetables.

Omega 6 fatty acids

The most important of these is linolenic acid, found in unrefined safflower, corn, sesame, and sunflower oils.

Our bodies can make all the fat needed for our daily metabolic processes except for these two essential fatty acids: Omega 3 and Omega 6.

Linolenic acid is converted to gamma-linolenic acid, which is found in evening primrose oil. Great claims have been made for the powers of evening primrose oil, especially for its success in treating PMS, and it is popularly believed to suppress menopausal flashing. Your intake of essential fat can be improved by including the following:

- Cold-pressed unrefined vegetable oils such as sesame and sunflower oil for salad dressing
- Extra virgin olive oil for cooking
- Oily fish, such as mackerel, sardines, etc.
- Nuts (almonds, pecans, brazil nuts, etc.) and seeds (sesame, pumpkin, sunflower, etc.)
- Tahini (creamed sesame seeds) for sauces and dressings
- Butter in moderation for spreading or cooking

On the go all the time

Pause for a moment and look at your body. It probably is relaxed and still. What you cannot see is energy machine inside that never rests and always is metabolically alive. This machine powers its operations mainly through the use of a basic sugar molecule called glucose. Your body *must* have glucose, and even under conditions of starvation, it will continue to obtain it as long as there is anything in your body that can be converted into glucose. All of the food you eat is broken down into glucose by way of the digestive system and absorbed through the wall of the intestines into the bloodstream. Once that happens, you have a high level of glucose in your blood— or high blood sugar.

AS THE BLOOD GLUCOSE RISES

As your blood sugar levels go up—as they do after eating simple carbohydrates such as a chocolate bar—your body has to make an instant decision. How much of that pure energy should be used for immediate needs, and how much should be stored for future requirements?

The instrument for this decision is the hormone insulin, which is produced by the pancreas and governs the chemistry of sugar in the body. A rise of sugar in the blood elicits a swift response from insulin, which quickly converts part of this glucose to glycogen, a starch that can be stored in muscles and the liver and that can be made readily available for energy use.

But what happens if all these glycogen areas are full and there is still more glucose in the blood than is needed that moment? In this case, insulin stimulates the conversion of the excess glucose to fat molecules called triglycerides: These are part of the overall profile of fats in the body and are often elevated in people with heart disease and diabetes.

THE ROLLER-COASTER GLUCOSE RIDE

Sadly, all those delicious sweet cakes, chocolates, and cookies are full of ingredients that are refined. The flour, for example, has been finely processed and the outer bran of the seed discarded. Most of the fiber is also removed. Fiber absorbs water and contributes to the growth of beneficial bacteria in your gut. This process makes a bulky stool, providing exercise for your bowel and keeping your intestine in healthy working order.

When you eat foods high in refined ingredients, digestion is very fast and glucose enters your body rapidly, causing your blood sugar levels to rise steeply. In addition, any food or drink that contains a stimulant, such as coffee, tea, alcohol, or chocolate, causes a sharp and rapid rise in blood glucose, which may make you feel temporarily more energetic. However, the effect is short-lived. Blood sugar levels soon slump again because simple carbohydrates are unable to maintain them.

When this happens, we feel tired and make a cup of tea or coffee, and eat a chocolate cookie. Presto! We are revived and full of energy once more. But this boost has caused blood sugar level to go up rapidly, thus repeating

the cycle of blood sugar swings. Over time, this roller-coaster stimulation exhausts the pancreas, so that it becomes unable to produce sufficient insulin to regulate blood sugar levels. The result is that too much glucose stays in the blood instead of being converted into energy or body fat.

If we have not eaten for three hours, blood glucose drops to quite a low level, and we again look for the quick boost. At the same time our adrenal glands make our livers produce more glucose. The combination of these two causes high levels of glucose in our blood, which again calls on the pancreas to overproduce insulin to reduce the glucose levels. The roller-coaster ride starts all over again, and our adrenal glands become exhausted because of repeated stimulation.

WHY SHOULD THIS MATTER WHEN I AM MENOPAUSAL?

There are many reasons why it is important to avoid the roller-coaster effect on blood sugar levels described above. Maintaining a steady blood sugar level can make a huge difference to how you feel emotionally and physically before, during, and after the menopause. Its imbalance puts you at risk of diabetes. And it is especially important during the menopausal years because of the effect on the adrenal glands. As described earlier (page 11), these glands convert androstenadione into estrone, which is the main source of estrogen after the menopause. The adrenal glands also produce a hormone called dehydroepiandrosterone (DHEA), which has been linked to a slowing of the aging process. It is therefore crucial that the adrenal glands are working to their optimum.

Since the maintenance of steady blood sugar levels is such an important factor during the menopause, it makes sense to modify or change your intake of food and drink accordingly. This will be of benefit for the rest of your life.

Looking East

In Japan, China, and Indonesia women so rarely experience hot flashes that their languages do not have words for this menopausal symptom. On the other hand, eight out of ten American women reportedly experience what are termed "power surges" or "hot flashes."

The explanation for this discrepancy, experts say, can be found in diet. The typical diet in the Far East is high in soy and, in Japan, low in processed and refined foods and high in mineral-rich seaweed and fresh fish oils. Not only do Japanese women eating a traditional diet have fewer incidences of hot flashes, they also have lower rates of breast cancer.

The rate of reported menopausal symptoms is also lower in other Asian women, although this could be attributed to a culture that raises its women to "Never complain, never explain." It has been noted that when Asian women move to the West and assume a Western diet, they rapidly develop the diseases encountered by Western women.

RECENT CHINESE STUDY

The China Diet Study began gathering information on the lifestyles of 6,500 adults in 1983. One hundred people from each of the 65 provinces comprising China answered 367 questions about their diets, lives, and bodies. This ten-year study is the most comprehensive investigation ever made of the eating habits of Chinese people.

It was an exacting, labor-intensive study, initially financed by the US National Cancer Institute, that could probably not have been done anywhere except China. Nowhere else is there a genetically similar population with such

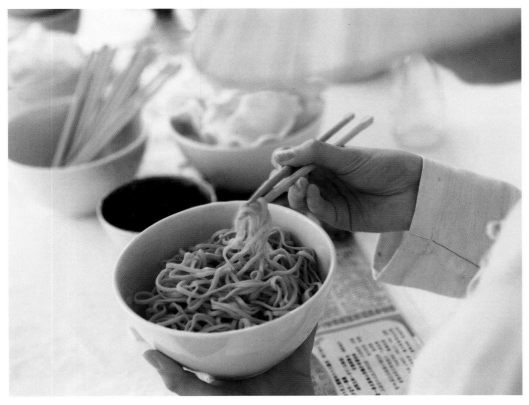

Far Eastern food is often low in processed and refined ingredients.

great regional differences in disease rates, dietary habits, and environmental exposures. And nowhere else could researchers afford to hire hundreds of trained workers to collect blood and urine samples and spend three days in each household gathering exact information on what and how much people ate, and then analyzing the food samples for nutrient content.

It was money well spent, for it has turned out to be a very important study—unique and well done, and challenges much of dietary dogma.

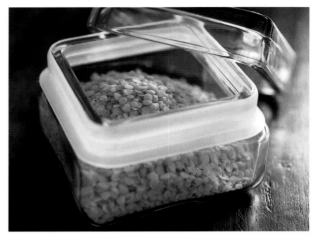
Legumes, such as lentils, contain phytoestrogens.

Highlights of this 920 page study show that:

- Chinese people consume 20 percent more calories than Americans do, but Americans are 25 percent heavier. This is because the Chinese eat three times the amount of starch and only one-third the amount of fat. This is a more important factor than exercise.
- Cholesterol levels in China are much lower than in the USA. The Chinese average is 127 mg/dL, compared with 212 mg/dL in the US.

Japanese diets are often high in mineral-rich seaweed.

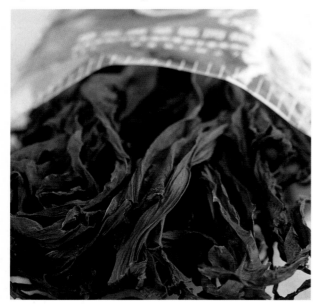

- Protein intake in China is one-third less than in the US—64 g (2¼ oz) per person per day, compared with 100 g (3½ oz).
- In China, mortality rates from colon cancer are lowest where cholesterol levels are lowest.
- For every heart attack in China, there are 16 in the United States.
- Female cancers relate to diet. A childhood diet high in protein, fat, calcium, and calories promotes rapid growth and early onset of menstruation. This increases a woman's risk for developing cancer of the reproductive organs and breast. Chinese women rarely get these cancers, and they begin menstruating 3 to 6 years later than American women.
- While Chinese women eat only half the calcium that American women eat, osteoporosis is uncommon in China. Most Chinese people eat no dairy products at all and obtain their calcium from plant sources.
- The Chinese diet is three times richer in fiber than the American diet, resulting in relatively low rates of colon cancer in China.
- Iron-deficiency anemia is rare in China, although their diet is mainly plant food and they eat less meat than in the West. The average Chinese

adult consumes twice the iron the average American does, and the vast majority of it comes from plants.

Soy far, so good

Some plants contain substances that, when eaten, can affect hormone status. These substances are called phytoestrogens.

Perhaps the most famous example of this is the soy bean. These beans contain phytoestrogens known as isoflavones, which make up about 75 percent of the soy protein. In the human gut, enzymes convert these into compounds that can have an estrogenic action, even though they are not hormones. Although the potencies are considerably weaker than the estrogen produced by the ovaries (estradiol), they appear to mimic and modulate estrogens and can help to stabilize hormone fluctuations. Depending on the tissue and the concentration, phytoestrogens either act as hormones or inhibit the actions of natural hormones. In this way, they may do a similar job as tamoxifen (the breast cancer drug), which binds onto estrogen receptors and inhibits breast cancer growth.

These are some of the foods that contain phytoestrogens:

- Wholegrains (such as wheat, corn, and oats)
- Legumes (such as chickpeas, mung beans, lentils, and peas)
- Garlic
- Flaxseed
- Sunflower and pumpkin seeds,
- Almonds, cashews, and peanuts
- Radishes
- Potatoes
- Fennel
- Celery
- Sprouting beans (such as alfalfa)
- Parsley
- Green tea
- Papaya
- Rhubarb
- Apples

However, it is the soy products like tofu (soy bean curd), tempeh, miso, tamari (wheat-free soy sauce made in the traditional way), natto, okara and yuba, as well as soy milk and soy protein powder, which are the simplest ways to incorporate phytoestrogens into your meals.

A recommended daily dose of 45 g (1½oz) of soy protein has been found to reduce hot flashes by 40 percent.

A slice of good fortune

Nearly 20 years ago, a woman living in Yorkshire, England, made a momentous decision, little knowing what would develop from it. Linda Kearns had been on hormone replacement therapy for 13 years following a hysterectomy and oophorectomy (removal of ovaries) but had never really felt 100 percent. She was always tired and a little under the weather. Following a breast cancer scare, she decided enough was enough and stopped taking HRT. Her hot flashes and night sweats reappeared overnight.

She began reading up about alternative remedies and discovered she could replace HRT with foods rich in phytoestrogens. The problem was that some natural seeds and grains on their own are rather unappetizing, so Linda set about creating a tasty cake.

A SLICE A DAY TO KEEP FLASHES AWAY

Within three weeks of starting to eat the resulting cake, her menopausal symptoms disappeared and she was bursting with energy. She now eats two slices of her cake every day at breakfast and after her evening meal.

When word got out, she found herself inundated with a request for the recipe (see right). Today, upwards of 2000 of these cakes (available in raisin, cherry, and cranberry), are baked every day at a Yorkshire bakery.

About 100 g (4 oz) a day (or a third of a 300 g [11 oz] cake) is usually adequate to deliver sufficient phytoestrogens to relieve menopausal symptoms. A 100 g slice looks generous, but it does not have to be eaten all at once. And you don't need to worry about the sugar and fat content: there are no added fats, other than those naturally occurring in the various seeds, and no added sugar.

Recipe for the Linda Kearns Cake

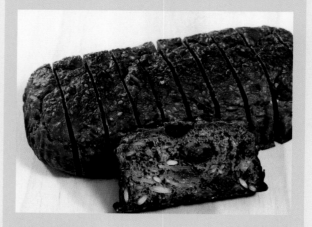

Ingredients

100 g (4 oz) soy flour	2 pieces of stem ginger, finely chopped
100 g (4 oz) wholewheat flour	200 g (8 oz) raisins
100 g (4 oz) oatmeal	750 ml (2½ cups) soy milk
100 g (4 oz) flaxseeds	1 tablespoon malt extract
50 g (2 oz) sunflower seeds	½ teaspoon nutmeg
50 g (2 oz) pumpkin seeds	½ teaspoon cinnamon
50 g (2 oz) sesame seeds	½ teaspoon ground ginger
50 g (2 oz) flaked almonds	

Place the dry ingredients in a large bowl and mix thoroughly. Add the soy milk and malt extract. Mix well and leave to soak for about 30 minutes. (If the mixture is too stiff, add more soy milk.) Spoon into two loaf pans lined with greaseproof paper and oil. Bake in the oven at 375°F/190°C for about 1¼ hours or until baked through. (Test for this with a skewer.) Turn out and leave to cool.

The cake is delicious with butter or spread. Ideally, eat a slice a day.

Note *The cake is not artificial HRT. It is a cake containing only the ingredients listed, which themselves contain natural plant phytoestrogens.*

Good health off the shelf

If you read glossy magazines, listen to commercial radio, or watch TV or if you explore the plethora of health websites on the Internet, you know that there is a thriving industry devoted to the promotion of vitamin and mineral supplements. These are aimed at people concerned about a variety of conditions, and combinations of vitamins and minerals increasingly are being marketed for specific groups of people, such as menopausal women.

Advertisements often feature an amazing display of attractively presented pills, potions, and packets, bristling with complicated neoscientific data on the labels. How do you decide which, if any of them, will improve or maintain your health?

First of all, you need to know what the various vitamins and minerals do in the human body.

VITAMINS

- **Vitamin A** maintains your healthy skin, eyes, bones, hair, and teeth.
- **Vitamin D** assists in the absorption and metabolism of calcium and phosphorus for strong bones and teeth.
- **Vitamin E** helps protect your red blood cells, circulation, and heart. As an antioxidant, vitamin E helps to protect cell membranes, fats, and vitamin A from destructive oxidation.
- **Vitamin K** is needed for proper clotting of your blood and is vital for bone formation.
- **Vitamin C** (ascorbic acid) is important for maintenance of your bones, teeth, collagen (which makes up 90 percent of our bone matrix), and blood vessels. We neither manufacture nor store our own vitamin C. It is water soluble and excreted within two or

RED BLOOD CELLS

Red cells float in the blood and are the means by which oxygen reaches all parts of the body. They contain a protein, hemoglobin, which has a special ability to grab oxygen molecules as the cells circulate through the lungs and then release the oxygen wherever it is needed in the tissues. Iron is an essential constituent of hemoglobin, and anemia is the result of lack of hemoglobin.

Pernicious anemia results not from lack of iron but from lack of Vitamin B_{12}.

three hours, so we need to make sure that we obtain adequate amounts daily.

Four of the B group vitamins—B_1, B_2, B_3, and B_6—release energy from the food we eat, as well as performing other functions.

- **Vitamin B_1** (thiamine) is needed for a normal appetite and for the functioning of a healthy nervous system.
- **Vitamin B_2** (riboflavin) is necessary for healthy skin and eyes.
- **Vitamin B_3** (niacin) helps to maintain the skin, nervous system, and proper mental functioning.
- **Vitamin B_6** plays a role in protein and fat metabolism and is essential for the function of red blood cells.
- **Vitamin B_5** (panthothenic acid) fights infections and strengthens the immune system.
- **Vitamin B_{12}** (cobalamin) prevents pernicious anemia and is necessary for a healthy nervous system.
- **Vitamin B_{17}** (amygdalin) is purported to control cancer.

MINERALS

- **Calcium** protects and builds bones and teeth and aids blood clotting.
- **Chromium** breaks down sugar for use in the body and helps to regulate blood pressure.
- **Iron** aids growth, promotes the immune system, and is essential for metabolism and production of hemoglobin.
- **Manganese** is needed for normal bone structure and is important for both the hormone production of the thyroid gland and for digestion.
- **Magnesium** is extremely important for the health of your bones, equally if not more important than calcium (see box, right). You need twice as much magnesium as calcium if the biochemistry of your bone formation is to run smoothly.
- **Phosphorus** maintains healthy, strong bones and teeth and is necessary for muscle and nerve function.
- **Potassium** regulates your body's water balance, aids muscle function and helps to dispose of the body's waste.

Spinach is a rich source of iron and vitamin K.

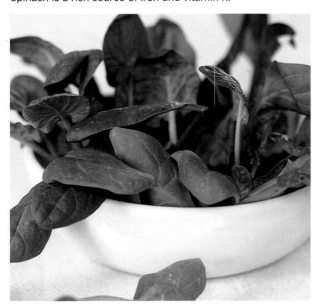

MARVELLOUS MAGNESIUM
Sixty percent of your body's magnesium stores are contained in your bones, particular the trabecular bone of your wrist, thighs, and vertebrae. Magnesium is vital in metabolizing calcium and vitamin C and helps to convert vitamin D to the active form necessary to ensure proper calcium absorption.

- **Selenium** is a trace element that occurs naturally in soil, food, and your body. It is a potent antioxidant, preventing or slowing aging, activating thyroid hormones, and keeping your liver functioning healthily.
- **Sulfur** helps to fight bacterial infection, aids your liver, and forms part of tissue-building amino acids.
- **Sodium** (salt) is essential for normal growth and helps muscles and nerve function. However, most people's diet contains too much sodium.
- **Zinc** is present in small amounts as a component of insulin and is required for blood sugar control, hearing, and taste. It is also important for wound healing and assists the activity of vitamin D in promoting the absorption of calcium.

The chart on page 118 to 121 shows what vitamins and minerals are available from various foods in your current diet. You might realize that you do not eat enough foods containing vitamins B_1 or B_{12}, or minerals such as magnesium or potassium, so increasing them with a supplement could be the answer. Equally, you may not like drinking milk or eating dairy products, so this chart will show you other foods from which you can gain calcium.

CALCIUM SUPPLEMENTS

If you decide to buy a calcium supplement, look very carefully at the label. Calcium carbonate is the cheapest and most widely marketed calcium supplement. It is otherwise known as chalk. Be aware that calcium carbonate is an inorganic mineral; it is mined from the ground and is not present in this particular form in any plant or animal. It can increase your risk of kidney stones and is not even particularly well absorbed into the body. On the other hand, calcium citrate is absorbed well. The following test will show you if the supplement you are taking is being absorbed: place your supplement in a glass of warm vinegar for 30 minutes, stirring every few minutes. The warm vinegar roughly represents the conditions found in your stomach. If the supplement does not dissolve after 30 minutes, try another type.

Sensible supplements

Supplements are regularly dismissed by nutritionists as being unnecessary. However, they may be the answer if you have neither the time nor inclination to prepare nutritious food or you are reassured by taking a tablet which contains a specified daily requirement. There is growing evidence that supplements can have a beneficial effect on menopausal symptoms.

Fatty acids

If you decide to take an appropriate vitamin and mineral preparation, the next most important nutritional group for long-range supplementation is the essential fatty acids. As mentioned earlier in this chapter, they are a vital component of every human cell, and your body needs them to:

- Insulate your nerve cells.
- Keep your skin and arteries supple.
- Balance your hormones.
- Keep you warm.

Flaxseeds provide a source of omega 3 fatty acids. Flaxseed oil is manufactured in either capsule form or lemon-flavored powder in 500 mg or 1,000 mg.

Flaxseeds can be bought as seeds or as oil.

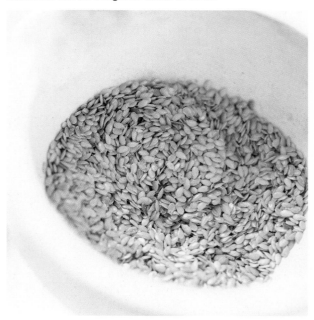

Food fitness

Try to buy high-quality food from reliable sources and eat:

- Fruits and vegetables – abundantly
- Wholegrains and cereals – moderately
- Bean, peas, and lentils – often
- Fats and concentrates (i.e., foods high in protein, fat, or sugar) – sparingly

The following foods are all rich sources of minerals and vitamins.

FRUIT

Apples *vitamins A, B₁, B₂, B₃, B₁₇, C, D, and E, iron, and manganese*

Apricots *sodium, zinc, and vitamin B₁₇*

Avocado *manganese, vitamins B, C, and E*

Bananas *potassium, chromium, vitamins B and C*

Blackberries *vitamins B, C, and E*

Cherries *vitamins B and C*

Cranberries *vitamin C*

Dates *sodium, vitamin B*

Figs *sodium, sulfur, vitamins B and C*

Grapefruit *potassium, phosphorus, vitamins B and C*

Grapes *Iron, vitamins B, C, and E*

Gooseberries *vitamins B, C, and E*

Guavas *vitamin C*

Kiwi fruit *vitamin C*

Lemon *vitamins B and C*

Loganberries *vitamins B and C*

Mangoes *vitamins B and C*

Melons *vitamin C*

Nectarines *zinc, vitamin B₁₇*

Olives *sodium*

Oranges *magnesium, vitamin C*

Papaya *vitamins A, B₁, B₃, B₅*

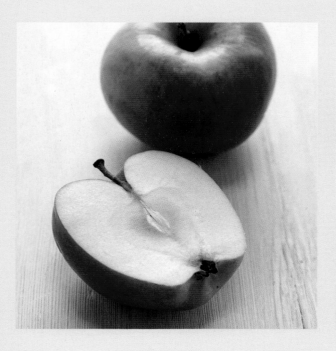

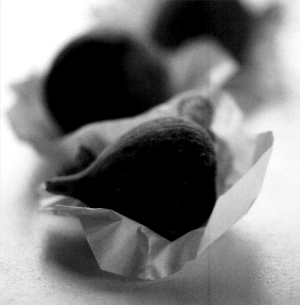

Passion fruit *vitamins B and C*

Peaches *manganese, vitamins B and C*

Pineapple *vitamin C*

Plums *iron, vitamins B17 and C*

Prunes *vitamins B and E*

Quince *iron, vitamins B and C*

Raspberries *sodium, sulfur, vitamins B, C, and E*

Rhubarb *vitamins B, C, and E*

Strawberries *sodium, sulfur, vitamins B and C*

Tomatoes *potassium, vitamins B, C and E*

Tangerines *vitamins B and C*

Ugli fruit (a citrus fruit indigenous to Jamaica, a cross between a grapefruit and a tangerine) *potassium, phosphorus, vitamin C, and magnesium*

VEGETABLES

Artichokes *potassium, vitamins A, B, and C*

Asparagus *potassium, vitamins A, B, C, and E*

Beans *vitamin B12*

Beets *vitamin C*

Broccoli *selenium, vitamin E*

Brussels sprouts *sulfur, vitamin C*

Carrots *sulfur, vitamin A, B, and C*

Cauliflower *potassium, vitamins B, C, and E*

Eggplant *magnesium and phosphorus, vitamin B*

Garlic *sulfur, vitamins A, B1, B2, B3, B5, and C*

Kale *calcium, phosphorus, potassium, sulfur, vitamin A*

Leafy green vegetables *iron, vitamins B2, C*

Mushrooms *vitamins C and E*

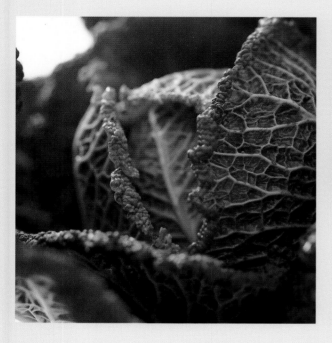

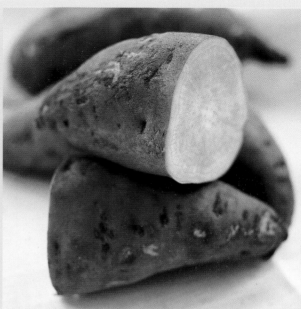

Okra *magnesium, sulfur, vitamins B and C*

Onions *selenium, sulfur, vitamins B$_3$ and C*

Parsley *vitamins A, B$_3$, B$_5$, and E*

Parsnips *sulfur, vitamins B, C, and E*

Peas *calcium, vitamins B and C*

Peppers *vitamin C*

Plantain *vitamins B and C*

Potatoes *calcium, chromium, sulfur, vitamin C*

Pumpkin *iron, zinc, vitamins B and C*

Radishes *potassium, vitamin C*

Red cabbage *magnesium, vitamins B and C*

Savoy cabbage *vitamins B, C, and E*

Spinach *calcium, iron chromium, vitamins B, E, and K*

Spring cabbage *vitamins B and C*

Spring onions *vitamin C*

Squash *iron, phosphorus*

Sweetcorn *vitamins B and E*

Watercress *vitamins B$_3$, C, and D*

White cabbage *vitamins B and C*

Yams (sweet potatoes) *vitamins A, B, and C*

Zucchini *vitamins B and E*

DAIRY FOOD

Butter *Enjoy occasionally.*

Cream *Resist!*

Cheese *vitamin B$_2$, enjoy in moderation, see the calcium chart*

Eggs *sodium, sulfur (egg yolk), zinc, vitamins B$_2$, B$_{12}$, and E*

Milk *vitamins B$_{12}$, D, and calcium*

Yogurt *vitamins A, B, D, and E*

MEAT, FISH AND SHELLFISH

Bacon *Buy the best! Grill rather than fry.*

Herring *vitamins B$_2$ and D*

Oysters *zinc, vitamin B*

Quahog (an edible clam) *phosphorus, selenium*

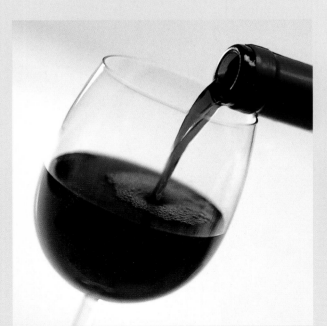

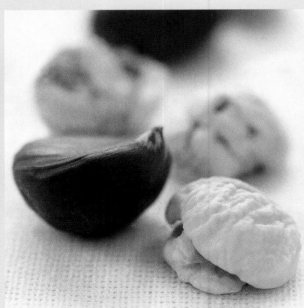

Salmon *calcium, vitamins B2 and D*
Tuna *phosphorus, selenium,
vitamins B2 and D*

BEANS

Chickpeas *vitamins C and E*
Soy beans *calcium, potassium*
Soy flour *vitamin B*

SEEDS

Pumpkin seeds *iron, zinc,
vitamins B and C*
Sesame seeds *calcium,
phosphorus, vitamin B1*
Sunflower seeds *vitamin B1*

NUTS

Almonds *calcium, magnesium,
vitamins B2 and E*
Brazil nuts *iron, phosphorus, vitamins
B and E*
Cashews *magnesium, vitamins B
and E*
Chestnuts *potassium, vitamins B and C*
Coconut *sulfur, vitamins B, C, and E*
Hazel nuts *vitamins B and E*
Peanuts *vitamin B1 and E*
Pecan *vitamins B and C*
Pine nuts *vitamin B*
Pistachio *vitamin B*
Walnuts *iron, magnesium,
vitamins B, C and E*

GRAINS AND CEREALS

BREAD

The staff of life. (Take care with some white
breads as they may contain sugar or dextrose
and/or flour improvers—the latter is fine if it
states "Ascorbic acid" on the label as this is a
form of vitamin C.)
Chapatis *vitamin B*

Rye bread *vitamins A, B1, B2, B3, B5,
B12, and E, and manganese*
Wholemeal bread *chromium and
manganese*

BREAKFAST CEREALS

(Read the label to check sugar content.)
Bran *selenium, phosphorus, iron,
vitamin B1*
Oats *magnesium, sodium,
vitamin B1*
Rice *iron, magnesium, phosphorus,
vitamin B1*
Wheatgerm *zinc, magnesium,
vitamins B1 and E*

BEVERAGES

Champagne *Enjoy!*
Cocoa *zinc, vitamins B and E*
Coffee *Reduce.*
Tea *manganese, vitamins B and C*
Water *Drink 8 glasses of water a day.*
Wine *Vitamin B is in red wine;
excellent for your heart!*

SWEET TREATS AND SAVORY SNACKS

Cakes *Resist!*
Chocolate *Special treat only!*
Cookies *Avoid; they are usually full of refined
sugar.*
Danish pastries *Resist!*
Honey *calcium*
Ice cream *calcium*
Jam *vitamin C*
Peanut butter *vitamins B, C, and E*
Potato chips *vitamins B, C, and E*
Sugar *Refined white has no vitamins,
molasses contains vitamin B.*

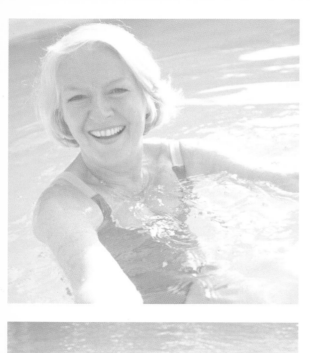
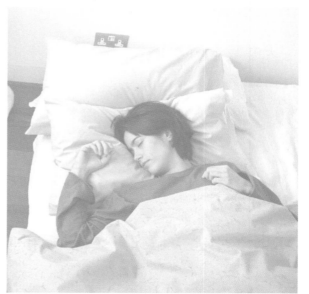
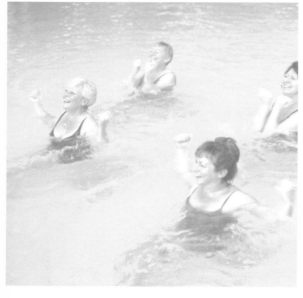
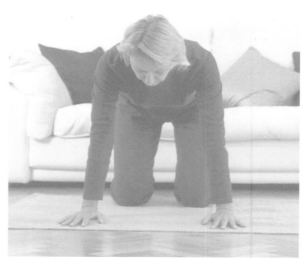
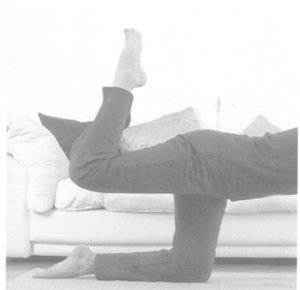
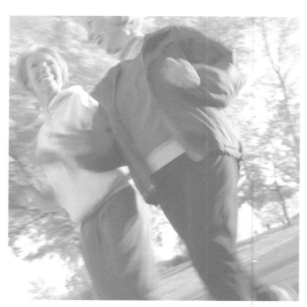

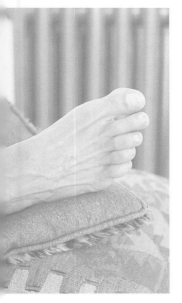

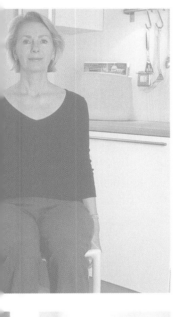

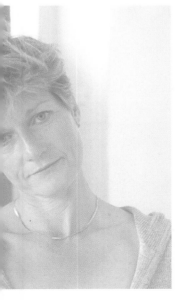

5

Get moving!

Exercise

The advantages of regular physical exercise are numerous and well-documented. Exercise allows us to burn fat efficiently and boosts our metabolism so that we continue to burn off calories at a faster rate, even after we have stopped exercising, thereby helping to control body weight.

Exercise can have a powerful all-round effect on your health. Regular exercise helps to keep the bowels working efficiently, which gets rid of waste products your body does not need.

In addition, it:

- Improves the function of the immune and lymph systems and the ability of the body to keep blood sugar levels in balance.
- Maintains bone density.
- Maintains muscle mass.
- Increases metabolism, burning calories and fat
- Reduces stress.
- Alleviates many menopausal symptoms, such as hot flashes.

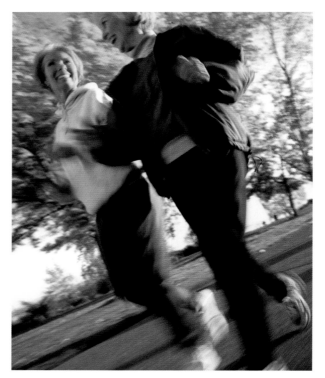

Exercising with a friend can be an extra motivation.

- Helps former smokers stay off cigarettes.
- Boosts the immune system, lessening vulnerability to colds and flu.
- Helps maintain flexibility and joint movement as you age.

COUNT THE CALORIES

How many calories do you burn off doing everyday activities? This is how much you can use up in 20 minutes:

Activity	Calories burned
Ironing	20
Housework	60
Digging the garden	100
Walking upstairs	120
Running upstairs	200

A healthy heart

Regular exercise is vital to keep your heart healthy. Research consistently shows that regular exercise keeps arteries flexible and reduces cholesterol levels.

Aerobic exercise, which speeds up your heart rate, is considered ideal for a healthy heart. Aim for 30 minutes of aerobic activity, such as swimming, brisk walking, running, and cycling, at least three times a week.

Start gently and build up gradually. Mild breathlessness is normal and healthy.

KEEPING UP THE PRESSURE

Physical activity can help to keep your blood pressure low. An hour of brisk walking five times a week is recommended for maximum benefit.

Build bones and muscles

Your bones and muscles need weight-bearing exercise to boost bone density. Try to include these activities into your exercise routine:

- Skipping
- Aerobics
- Tennis
- Running
- Gentle weight-training

Exercise your mind

Your mental health also benefits from regular exercise. Physical activity releases "feel-good" endorphins, which boost your mood and help you relax.

Swimming and jogging can also help calm your mind, while your mood often is lifted by steps accompanied by music. Dancing is guaranteed to banish the blues of a difficult menopause (see page 138).

ENDORPHINS
Endorphins are chemicals secreted by the brain to help us to feel happier, more alert, and calmer.

Getting motivated

Going to a gym or health fitness center may suit you and your lifestyle—but it may not. Many of us are put off by the membership fees and the need to buy the right gear, as well as by worrying about our exposure in front of strangers. It is easy to feel intimidated or uncomfortable, and you soon lose your motivation if you don't enjoy the experience.

But many gyms and leisure centers offer a huge range of possibilities—from salsa and belly dancing to kickboxing and rockclimbing. It is worth taking the time to investigate what is available.

Swimming is a fun way to exercise.

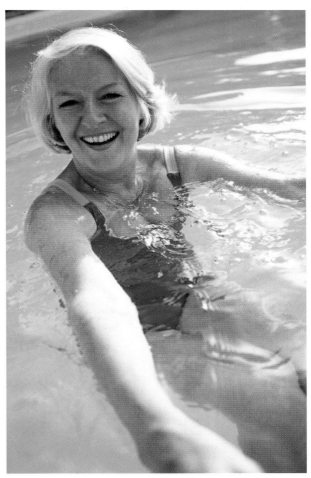

leg swing

This exercise will improve your flexibility and circulation. Use a mat if you find your joints are uncomfortable when kneeling on the floor.

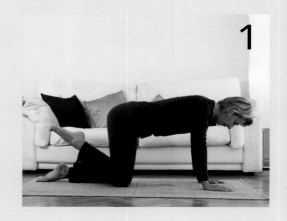

1 Kneel on all fours. You can do this exercise with or without small hand weights. If you choose to use them, place one in the bend of your right knee. Lift you lower leg slightly to keep the weight in place.

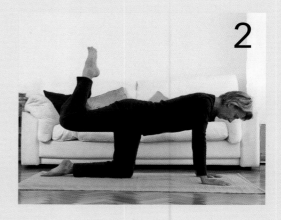

2 Lift the bent knee until it is level with your spine and your right foot is pointing up to the ceiling.

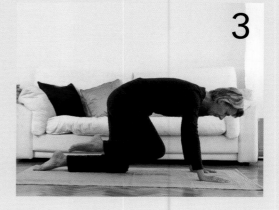

3 Swing your bent leg down and through until your knee is under your chest. Return it to the starting position and lower to the ground. Repeat the exercise using the other leg.

kneeling hand walk

This exercise places much needed pressure on your hand and arm joints and bones. Make sure that your spine is kept straight by not letting your head hang.

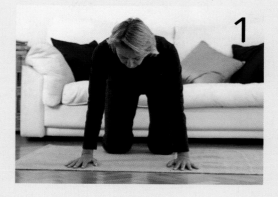

1 Kneel down on all fours, keeping your back straight.

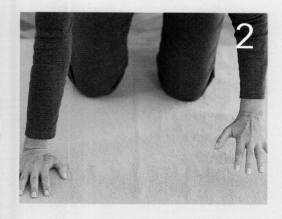

2 Keeping your knees and feet still, slowly walk your hands forward until your arms are carrying much of your weight. Be sure to keep your spine straight.

3 Now walk your hands out to the side. This will greatly increase the strength of the bones in your arms. Then walk your hands back in the reverse pattern until you are kneeling comfortably, balanced on all fours again. Repeat this a few times and then stand up.

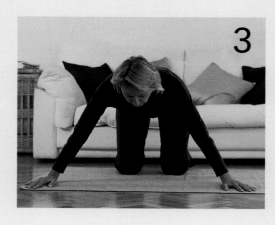

Posturing with purpose

In childhood we have a naturally relaxed posture, but as we mature our bodies start to reflect the strains of life. It is easy to get into the habit of slouching in a soft lounge chair or sitting hunched in front of a computer screen without a break. Some jobs necessitate standing for long periods or performing repetitive actions. All these occupations can place undue stress on specific parts of our bodies.

Every day we acquire incorrect posture without noticing that it is happening. This in turn filters through to other physical functions and depletes our energy.

Other postural problems can have an emotional basis. People who carry an emotional burden can often be seen to literally carry it on their shoulders.

One condition that can be rectified by particular exercises is kyphosis. This curvature of the top of the spine is sometimes associated with osteoporosis and is therefore often seen in postmenopausal women.

If kyphosis is becoming a problem for you, you may find it helpful to make the Pilates system part of your daily routine. This exercise system was formulated by Joseph Pilates, a German gymnast, skier, boxer, wrestler, and physical fitness trainer. It is based on the premise that our physical movements most benefit our health when they are conscious actions serving our will. So whether we are walking, sitting, turning, or stretching, we should always direct our movements, making it clear in our minds as to exactly what we are doing and how advantageous it will be to us.

Pilates is different from other forms of exercise primarily because of its holistic approach and its combined training

of mind and body to achieve correct postural alignment. Its key elements are:

- Lengthening short muscles and strengthening weak muscles.
- Improving the quality of movement.
- Focusing on the core postural muscles to stabilize the body.
- Working to place the breath correctly.
- Controlling even the smallest movements.
- Understanding and improving good body mechanics.
- Mental relaxation.

BAD POSTURE   GOOD POSTURE

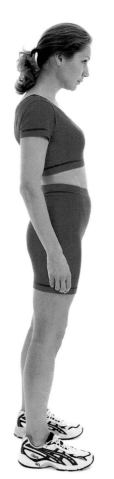
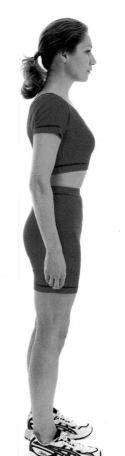

Good posture is not just about having a straight back. It lends balance to our limbs, allowing movements such as walking to be performed more smoothly. We all have our own unique way of walking, and an awareness of your body's posture can add balance and control to these otherwise unconscious movements, whether walking, standing, sitting, or lying.

Standing

If you watch people standing—say at a bus stop, on a station platform, in a check-out line—you notice how often they simply do not know what to do with their bodies.

They put the weight on one leg, bending the other, then shift their weight to the other leg. There is an attempt to stand up straight, but knees get locked and the pelvis is pushed forward, creating an exaggerated hollow in the lower spine. And as for arms, we often do not know what to do with them! Arms may be folded across our bodies, hands may be clasped behind our backs, or we may fidget with our clothes, purse, or briefcase. It is as if we have no sense of gravity within our bodies. If we can find it, it will hold us in a position of balance and ease.

HOW TO STAND

- Stand with your feet hip-width apart.
- Make sure that both your legs face forward.
- Your legs need to be straight, but your knees should not be locked back into the joint.
- Allow your arms to rest naturally at your sides, falling over the middle of your hips.
- Feel your weight being supported by the middle of each foot.
- Do not rock back, allowing the heels to take your weight, or place your weight on the balls of your feet.

It is important to learn how to stand with good posture.

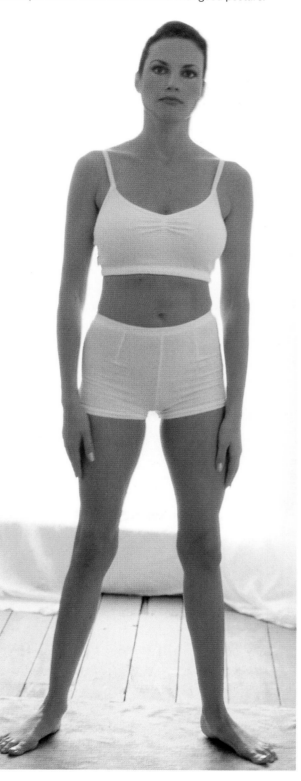

Once you have achieved this way of resting with your muscles relaxed and your balance centered you will find that you tire less easily, feel taller, and are more relaxed in your environment.

Sitting

Like standing, sitting is something we often do not do very well. We sit balanced on one hip bone, then we shift to the other. We cross our legs or sit with one leg underneath us. We wriggle around in our seats, trying to find a position that is comfortable. When we eventually do find a comfortable position, it does not seem to last long.

We try to find external solutions to this, such as lumbar supports on chairs or car seats. The trouble with these is that they are not suitable for most of us; they are too low down to give support where it is needed. Instead, they tend to push the lumbar spine forward, and this in turn can push the abdominal muscles and the internal organs forward.

CHOOSING A CHAIR

When looking for a chair that will properly support the back and allow you to adopt a good sitting posture, you need to check out the following:

- You should be able to sit comfortably with your whole thigh supported by the seat of the chair.
- You should be able to place both feet flat on the floor comfortably.
- The back support should be as high as your shoulder blades. The backs of many office chairs are either lower or higher than this.

Remember to sit with your weight evenly distributed, your knees slightly apart in order to support the weight, and your feet together, underneath your knees.

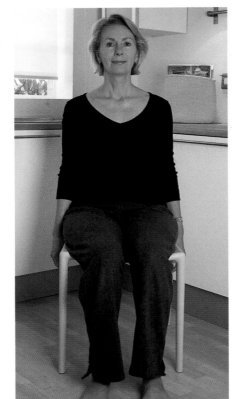

You should be able to place both feet flat when you sit down.

Lying down

We spend about a third of each day lying down. Again, we do not give much thought to this, we just do it. And because we are sleeping for much of this time, we are unaware of our position.

Lying down should be our ultimate position of rest, but still we manage to contort ourselves in various ways that put strain on our muscles and limit our blood circulation. How often have you awakened with stiff muscles and a sore back? Sleeping on your stomach does not support your spine, which often gets twisted if one leg is bent up when you are in this position. To breathe properly while lying on your stomach, your head has to be turned to one side. This not only twists the neck but can also trap nerves in it, leading to feelings of numbness or "pins and needles" during sleep or waking.

The best positions for sleeping are either on your back or side. If you have a lower-back problem, it can be helpful to sleep with a pillow between your knees.

Wake-up time!

How often do you wake up and instinctively feel the need for a good stretch, even before you put a foot out of bed? Quite often your whole body moves into that stretch, elongating your back, arms, and legs, but without you consciously willing them to move. You might even yawn while you do it—another reflex action. Stretching your body like this feels pleasurable, but how good is it for you?

Stretching helps to lengthen your muscles and relax them. If we think of our muscles as having the same qualities as elastic bands, it is easy to understand the aim of doing stretches. Too much tension tightens our

muscles and makes us feel tired and depressed. Relieving the muscle tension by stretching brings back elasticity and aids muscle and joint harmonization.

Tight muscles cause a number of problems. Because muscles are interconnected, an injury may not arise in the area of tightness, but instead in an area connected to it. For instance, lower back injuries can result from tight hamstring muscles at the back of the knees. Tight hamstrings restrict mobility and result in your lower back also being tight. Very tight hamstrings pull on your pelvis, creating postural problems.

Stretching your muscles should feel comfortably uncomfortable. The sensation should be one of stretching, not one of tearing. Take care! If you experience a hot, shooting pain while stretching then stop the exercise immediately. Otherwise you are likely to cause damage.

While you sleep you will change your position many times.

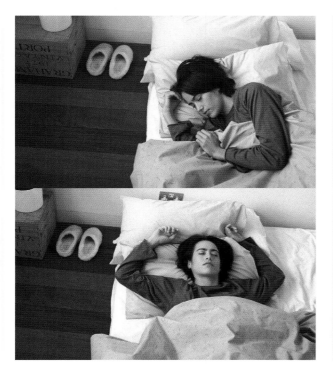

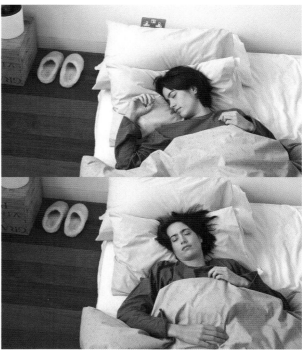

hamstring stretch

The hamstrings are the two tendons at the rear of the hollows of your knees. Tendons are constructed of tough, inelastic fibrous tissue that connects a muscle with its bony attachment. This pilates exercise will help you to stretch them.

1 Place your buttocks on the edge of a desk or the arm of a sofa, just enough to support your pelvis. Place the heel of one foot on a low stool in front of you. Make sure that the stool is close enough for you not to have to stretch your leg out to reach it. Turn your foot outward to stretch your buttock and hamstring muscles.

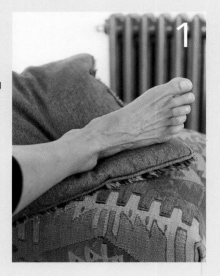

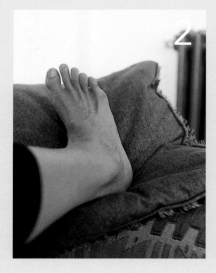

2 Next, turn your foot inward to stretch the inner part of your hamstring.

shoulder stretch

This is a pilates exercise that will help you to stretch your shoulders. Repeat this exercise 3 to 6 times.

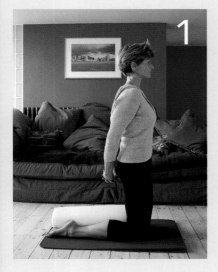

1 Kneel with a cushion between your knees and calves. Squeeze the cushion and clasp your hands behind your back at the level of your buttocks. Breathe in, pull up your pelvic floor and pull in your stomach muscles.

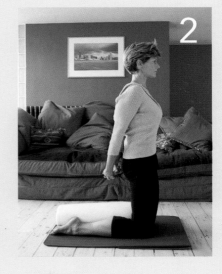

2 Breathe out, pull your shoulders back and squeeze your shoulder blades together.

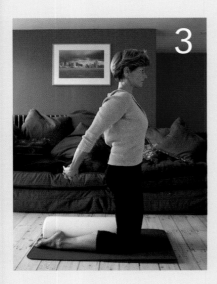

3 Stretch your clasped hands away from your buttocks. Hold the position for 3 breaths.

neck stretch

The aim of this pilates exercise is to stretch and relax your neck muscles. Repeat each of these steps 1 to 3 times.

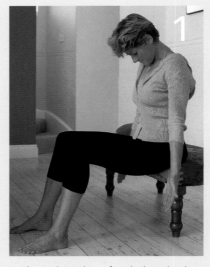

1 Sit on the edge of a chair or bed. Tuck your chin in toward your chest. Allow yourself to melt like an ice cube from your chest and stomach muscles, letting the spine drop forward. Hold the position for 10 to 30 long slow breaths.

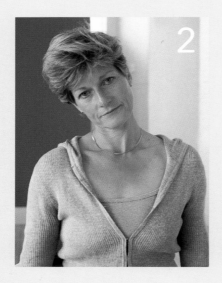

2 Drop your right ear toward your right shoulder as far as it is comfortable. Hold for 10 to 30 long slow breaths.

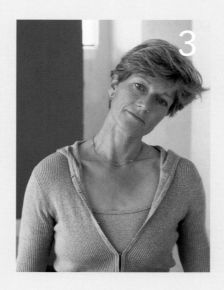

3 Now drop your left ear toward your left shoulder as far as it is comfortable. Hold for 10 to 30 long slow breaths.

cat stretch

This exercise will help to increase your spinal articulation.
Repeat this exercise 3 to 6 times.

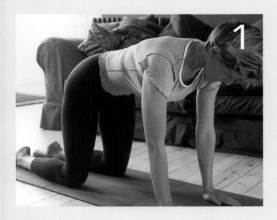

1 Start on your hands and knees, making sure that your hands are beneath your shoulders and that your hips are above your knees. Make sure that your back is flat and that your head and neck are in alignment with your back, parallel to the floor. Breathe in, sensing the breath coming in between your shoulder blades. Pull up your pelvic floor and pull in your stomach muscles.

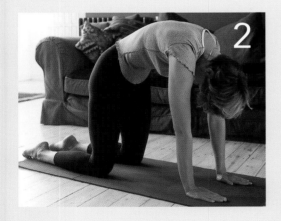

2 Breathing out, curl your tailbone underneath you, push into your hands and lift your breastbone, tucking your chin and then your head underneath. Hold this position and breathe in. Breathe out and lower yourself back into the starting position (step 1) by reversing the sequence, bringing your head back up to its position parallel with the floor, followed by your chin and tailbone.

Get fit without the fuss!

There are many ways for you to introduce more exercise into your lifestyle without making big changes.

- If your workplace is close to your home, you could get up a little earlier, leave your car at home, and walk to work. You will be doing your bit for the environment that way as well!
- If you have a longer journey, get off the subway, bus, or train two stops earlier. A brisk 20 minute walk each day is excellent for getting your heart pumping, and you will feel refreshed and energized when you start work.
- Housework and gardening can both help you work up a sweat: push the vacuum that much harder, rake the lawn more energetically, and stretch up with that feather duster. It all makes a difference!
- Get into the habit of taking a lunchtime stroll.

Just walking to the sandwich shop will boost your fitness levels and help you avoid that post-lunchtime energy slump.
- If you work at home, it is theoretically easier to take a break, but in practice you need to discipline yourself to build in time for exercise. It helps to have a dog—dogs always want to go for walks!
- Alternatively, you could exercise at home in front of an exercise video.
- If sexual intimacy is part of your life, vigorous sex can be a great form of exercise, boosting your heart rate, increasing your lung capacity, and giving your muscles a workout. However, sex may be the last thing on your mind until your menopausal symptoms are under control, and an understanding partner can make all the difference.
- If you are spending the day shopping, try walking between shopping areas, rather than jumping on the bus or in the car. Carrying bags is a good way to combine a walk with weight-bearing exercise.
- When you are shopping in a department store,

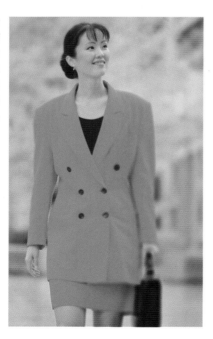

Walking to work, or walking for part of your journey, is an easy way to increase the amount of exercise you do each day.

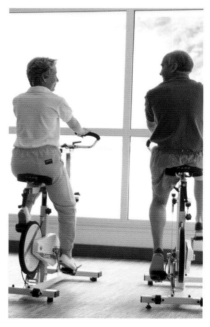

If you don't want to join an exercise class, try visiting your local gym and using their exercise machines.

take the stairs instead of the elevator or escalator. Climbing stairs helps tone your leg muscles and increases your heart rate.

- Stretch, skip, and jog for 5 to 10 minutes while you are watching the TV or listening to music.

Some common sense precautions when starting to exercise

- If you are over 50 and have health risk factors or have been extremely inactive, see your doctor before starting an exercise program.
- Exercise must be regular. A weekend blitz— where your usual sedentary self suddenly leaps into six hours of tennis—is more dangerous than helpful.
- Stop if you feel short of breath, a muscle strain, joint pain, or numbness and tingling, especially in your chest and arms.
- Use the right shoes. Exercise has become shoe-specific, with walking shoes for walking, step shoes for step aerobics, and many kinds of running and aerobic dance shoes. You may be tempted to use the same pair for every activity, but an investment in proper shoes is essential— for the sake of your feet!
- Do not overlook the importance of sleep. If you are suffering menopausal night sweats, your sleeping pattern will be totally out of kilter. It is important to try to catch up on sleep as and when you are able to.
- If you need some instruction, get it. Books and videos can give you an idea on how to get started, but if you want to go past the basics, join a class.
- Drink a glass of water before and after exercising. Do not rely on thirst as an indicator of how much water you need. If you are thirsty, you are already water-depleted.
- Sports such as golf and tennis are fun and a

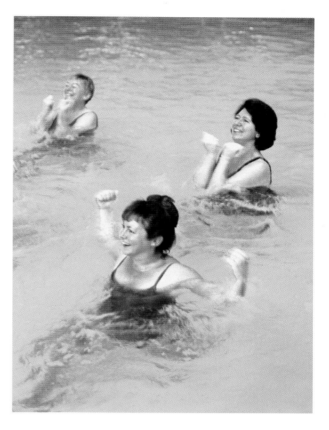

Find out about local exercise classes, You may be surprised at the amount of activities you can join in.

great way to socialize. However, because the nature of these sports require you to constantly start and stop, they rarely keep your heart rate consistently high enough to qualify as aerobic exercise.

- If you want to build your stamina and maintain a healthy heart, choose continuous-movement activities such as walking, swimming, or aerobic dancing.

SHOULD I EXERCISE WHEN I FEEL ILL?

If you have a headache or stuffy nose or you are sneezing, try exercising for 10 minutes, then evaluate how you feel. If you feel fine, continue. But if you have a chesty cough, stomach pain, or muscle strain it's best to skip your exercise session a day or two.

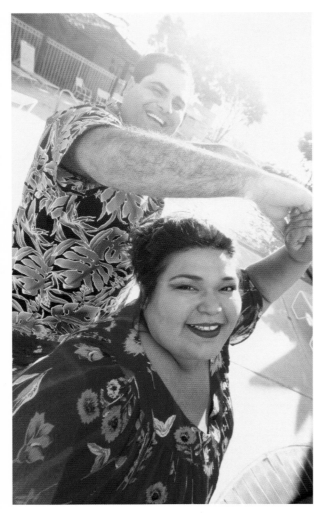

If you don't want to join your local gym, why not try dancing lessons instead.

Let's dance!

You may have vacationed abroad and returned with glowing memories of cultures in which dance is a vital part of life.

And what a choice we have worldwide! Where once social dancing was restricted to the traditional ballroom, nowadays clubs offering instruction in flamenco, lambada, line-dancing, and breakaway swing (jiving plus a few solo moves) have sprung up all over the place, with salsa and Argentine tango particularly on the rise.

Dancing is an instinctive celebration of our physical state of life: We do it when we feel good, and we feel good when we do it. Dancing puts us in touch with ourselves and with others; the touch of another person confirms we are real and alive.

An evening's dancing as is as good a form of exercise as a three-hour hike. Dancing:

- Releases energy and emotion.
- Pumps blood up our legs, which is good for our hearts.
- Keeps our brains tuned.
- Promotes supple posture and relaxation.
- Encourages self-confidence and a sense of achievement as we master a new skill.
- Gives us the opportunity to get up close and personal with a range of partners in a setting where ability and enthusiasm transcend age, gender, and class.

Whatever your choice of exercise—enjoy it! If the "feel-good" factor is missing, then try something different.

Nobody cares if you can't dance well. Just get up and dance. Great dancers are not great because of their technique; they are great because of their passion.

MARTHA GRAHAM,
US dancer and teacher (1895–1991)

Bibliography

Chapter 1

Booth, M., Beral, V., and Smith, P. *Risk factors for ovarian cancer: a case control study.*
British Journal of Cancer 60,
May 1989.

Celso-Ramon, Garcia, and Berg Cutler, Winnifred. *Preservation of the ovary: a reevaluation. Fertility and Sterility.*
The American Fertility Society 42(4),
October 1984.

Ford, G. *Listening to your Hormones.*
Prima, 1996.

Green, A., et al. *Tubal sterilisation, hysterectomy and decreased risk of ovarian cancer.*
International Journal of Cancer 71,
1997, pp. 948–951.

Loft, A., et al. *Incidence of ovarian cancer after hysterectomy: a nationwide controlled follow-up.*
British Journal of Obstetrics and Gynaecology 104(11), 1997,
pp. 1296–1301.

Mason, A. *Health and Hormones.*
Penguin Books, 1960.

Melville, A. *Natural Hormone Health.*
Thorsons, 1990.

Sellman, S. *Hormone Heresy.*
Getwell International, 2000.

Teaff, N. and Wiley, K.
Perimenopause – preparing for the change.
Prima, 1999.

Yaegashi, N. et al. *Incidence of ovarian cancer in women with prior hysterectomy in Japan.*
Gynaecology and Oncology 68(3),
1998, pp. 244–246.

Chapter 2

Beckham, N. *The wild yam scam: when not to believe the unbelievable.*
Townsend Letter for Doctors and Patients, Feb–March 2002.

Clark, J. *Hysterectomy and the Alternatives.*
Virago, 1993; Vermilion, 2000.

Coney, S. *The Menopause Industry.*
Spinifex Press, Australia, 1991.

Day, L. et al. *Randomised factorial trials of falls prevention among older people living in their own homes.*
British Medical Journal 325, 2002,
p.128.

Dibba, B., et al. *Bone metabolism.*
American Journal of Clinical Nutrition 71, 2000, pp. 544–549.

DiSaia, P.J., and Brewster, W.R. *Hormone replacement therapy for survivors of breast and endometrial cancer.*
Current Oncology Reports 4, 2002,
pp. 152–158.

Duvernoy, C.S., and Mosca, L. *Hormone replacement therapy trials: an update.*
Current Atherosclerosis Reports 4,
2002, pp. 156–160.

Felson, T., et al. *The effect of postmenopausal estrogen therapy on bone density in elderly women.*
New England Journal of Medicine 329, 1993, pp. 1141–1149.

Fogelman, I. *Screening for osteoporosis.*
British Medical Journal 391, 1999,
pp. 1148–1149.

Gennazini, A.R. *Hormone Replacement Therapy and Cardiovascular Disease: the current status of research and practice.*
Parthenon, 2002.

Grodstein, F., et al. *Postmenopausal hormone use and risk for colorectal cancer and adenoma.*
Annals of Internal Medicine 128,
1998, pp. 705–712.

Hulley, S., Grady, et al. *Randomised trial of estrogen and progesterone for secondary prevention of coronary heart disease in post-menopausal women.*
Journal of the American Medical Association 280, 1998, pp. 605–613.

Kenton, L. *Passage to Power.*
Vermilion, 1996.

Key, T., et al. *Dietary habits and mortality in 11,000 vegetarians and health-conscious people: results of a 17 year follow up.*
British Medical Journal 313, 1996, pp. 775–779

Kivipelto, M., et al. *Midlife vascular risk factors and Alzheimer's disease in later life.*
British Medical Journal 332: 2001, pp. 1447–1451.

Lee J.R. *Is natural progesterone the missing link in osteoporosis prevention and treatment?*
Medical Hypotheses 35, 1991, pp. 314–318.

Lee JR. *Osteoporosis reversal – the role of progesterone.*
International Clinical Nutrition Review 10(3), July 1990.

Michels, K.B. *The contribution of the environment (especially diet) to breast cancer risk.*
Breast Cancer Research 4, 2002, pp. 58–61.

Morrisey, D., et al. *Management of the climacteric. Postgraduate Medicine 108(1),* 2000.

Mosca, L., et al. *Hormone replacement therapy and cardiovascular disease. A Statement for healthcare professionals from the American Heart Association.*
Circulation 104, 2001, p. 499.

Murphy, S., et al. *Milk consumption and bone mineral density in middle aged and elderly women.*
British Medical Journal 308, 1994, pp. 939–941.

Prentice, A. *Osteoporosis.*
Proceedings of the Nutrition Society 56, 1997, pp. 357–367.

Purdie, D., and Crawford, I. *Management of the symptomatic menopause.*
Pharmaceutical Journal 263(7070), 1999, pp. 750–753.

Ridley, M. Genome – *The autobiography of a species in 23 chapters.*
Fourth Estate, 1999.

Schairer, C., et al. *Estrogen-progestogen hormone replacement therapy associated with greater increase in breast cancer risk than therapy with estrogen alone.*
Journal of the American Medical Association 283, 2000, pp. 485–491.

Shifren, J., et al. *Transdermal testosterone treatment in women with impaired sexual function after oophorectomy.*
New England Journal of Medicine 343, 2000, pp. 682–688.

Thomas, T. *A role for estrogen in the primary prevention of Alzheimer's disease.*
Climacteric 4, 2001, pp. 102–109.

Chapter 3

Bradford, N. *The Hamlyn Encyclopaedia of Complementary Health.*
Hamlyn, 2000.

Eden, J. *Herbal medicines for menopause: do they work and are they safe?*
Medical Journal of Australia 174, 2001, pp. 63–64.

Feder, G., and Katz, T. *Randomised controlled trials for homoeopathy.*
British Medical Journal 324, 2002, pp. 498–499 (Editorial).

Glenville, M. *Natural Alternatives to HRT.*
Kyle Cathie, 1997.

Israel, D., and Youngkin, E. *Herbal therapies for perimenopausal and menopausal complaints.*
Pharmacotherapy 17(5), 1997, pp. 970–984.

Oleson, T., and Flocco, W. Randomized controlled study of premenstrual symptoms treated with ear, hand and foot reflexology. *American Journal of Obstetrics and Gynecology. 82(6),* December 1993.

Roland, P. *How to Meditate.* *Hamlyn,* 2000.

Simonton, O.C. *Getting Well Again.* *Bantam Books* 1978.

Whiteaker, S. *The Good Retreat Guide.* *Rider,* 2001.

Wiegnand, M. *A gentle alternative in the therapy of perimenopausal symptoms.* *Biology Therapy X11(1),* 1994.

Chapter 4

Atkins, R. *Dr Atkins New Diet Revolution.* *Vermilion,* 1992.

Cooke, B. *Nutritional supplements in herbal practice.* *European Journal of Herbal Medicine 3,* 1997.

Davis, S. *Phytoestrogen therapy for menopausal symptoms?* *British Medical Journal 323,* 2001, pp. 354–355.

Diehl, Hans. *Huge diet study indicts fat and meat.* *Lifeline Health Letter* September-October 1990 (discussion of the China Diet Study).

Husband, A. *Phytoestrogens and menopause.* *British Medical Journal 32A,* 2002, pp. 52.

Mayo Clinic. *Soy and hot flashes: more heat than substance?* www.MayoClinic.org, 2000.

Mervyn, L. *The Dictionary of Vitamins.* *Thorsons,* 1984.

Norman, J. *Aromatic Herbs.* *Dorling Kindersley,* 1989.

Oliwenstein, L. *That certain age.* *Vegetarian Times* July 1999.

Savarin-Brillat, J.A. *The Physiology of Taste.* *Penguin,* 1970 (first published 1825).

Chapter 5

Blount, T., and McKenzie, E. *Pilates System.* *Hamlyn,* 2001.

Index

Acknowledgements

Acknowledgements in Source Order

Acestock Ltd 22 bottom left, 41, 58.

Alamy/Phoebe Dunn 8-9 bottom right, 14, /Image Source 2 center, 7, 22 center, 28, /Imagestate 122 top center, 131, /Peter Mumford 68-69 bottom right, 93.

Bubbles/Jennie Woodcock 57.

Getty Images/Samuel Ashfield 37, /Ron Chapple 8 center, /Chris Cheadle 103, /Jim Cummins 2 top left, 48, /Candice Farmer 2-3 top right, 122 center left, 137, /Howard Grey 8 bottom center, 13, /David Hanover 87, /Walter Hodges 122 bottom center, 124, /Romilly Lockyer 122 top left, 125, /Stuart McClymont 2 bottom center, 138, /Laurence Monneret 8-9 top right, 18, 22 top left, 24, /Antony Nagelmann 68 center, 102, /Andreas Pollok 68-69, 88, /Anne Rippy 8 bottom left, 65, /Mark Scott 104–105 center right, 106, /Steve Smith 56, /V.C.L. 27, /Terry Vine 8 center left, 15, /Mel Yates 100.

Octopus Publishing Group Limited/Colin Bowling 2 bottom left, 62, 77, 82 center left, 82 bottom right, /Colin Bowling /Organon Laboratories Ltd. 23 bottom right, 30, 32 center right, 34 left, /Colin Bowling / Pharmacia Corporation 34 right, /Colin Bowling /Schering Health Care Ltd. 22 center left, 31 center right, /Jean Cazals 105 top center, 120 left, /Colin Gotts 129, /Sandra Lane 104 top right, 116, /Sean Myers 83, /Peter Pugh-Cook 3 center right, 9 center right, 10, 23 top right, 59, 68 bottom left, 94, 97, 128 left, 128 right, /William Reavell 2 top center, 2 center left, 23 center right, 60, 92, 101, 104 top left, 104 center left, 104 center, 104 bottom left, 104 bottom center, 105 bottom right, 107, 108 right, 111, 112 top, 117, /Gareth Sambidge 66, 68 center left, 69 center right, 95 top left, 95 center right, 95 bottom left, /Nikki Sianni 8 top left, 70, 90, 122 center, 122 bottom left, 123 center right, 126 top, 126 center, 126 bottom, 127 center left, 127 top right, 127 bottom right, 130, /Ian Wallace 3 bottom right, 68 top center, 91, 99 top, 99 center, 108 left, 112 bottom, 118 left, 118 right, 119 left, 120 right, /Philip Webb 119 right, /Mark Winwood 123 top right, 123 bottom right, 132 top right, 132 bottom left, 133 top left, 133 center right, 133 bottom left, 134 center left, 134 top right, 134 bottom center, 135 top left, 135 bottom right.

Image State 136 left.

Science Photo Library/David Gifford 50, /Tim Malon & Paul Biddle 74, /Jerry Mason 32 bottom right, /Andrew McClenaghan 75, /Will & Deni McIntyre 22 top center, 46, /Professors P.M. Motta & J. Van Blerkom 8 top center, 17, /Perlstein, Jerrican 1, 136 right, /Sinclair Stammers 22 center bottom, 44, /Tek Image 68 top left, 72, /Sheila Terry 31 bottom right, 68 bottom center, 78, /Th Foto-Werbung 79, /Jim Varney 55, /Hattie Young 61.

Wellfoods Limited/tel: +44 (0) 1226 381 712/ www.bake-it.com 114.